THE FOOD JUNGLE

Your Guide
To Healthy Eating

Nancy and Eduardo Balingasa

First Edition

(PM) Printed Matters. The Woodlands, Texas

Published by: (PM) Printed Matters
114 Sage Blue Court
The Woodlands, Texas 77382-1347
(409) 273-2943; (888) 273-3155
Fax: (409) 273-6943
Email: info@printedmatters.com
Web: http://www.printedmatters.com

Book Design, Cover, and
  Illustrations by: Edu Balingasa, Jr.

Publisher's Cataloging-in-Publication
(Provided by Quality Books, Inc.)

Balingasa, Nancy
    The food jungle : your guide to healthy eating /
    Nancy and Eduardo Balingasa.
    -- 1st ed.
    p. cm.
    LCCN: 99-90856
    ISBN: 0-9672087-0-X

    1. Nutrition--Popular works. 2. Food--Health
aspects--Popular works. 3. Food additives.
I. Balingasa, Eduardo. II. Title.

RA784.B35 1999   613.2
                    QB199-1151

To

Cesareo and Carrie Gaane;
Anthony, John Stephen, Carrie, and
Patrick Faustino; and Edu Balingasa, Jr.

TABLE OF CONTENTS

APPENDICES:

INTRODUCTION

This is **YOUR SURVIVAL KIT** in the food jungle

How This Book Can Help You

The authors seek to inform and explain to the reader what one needs to know about harmful food ingredients, food labels, essential nutrients, and other topics related to food shopping and healthy eating. All these information will be the reader's tool in making the right decisions on what foods to buy. Look inside this book for:

➤ A list of food additives that can cause harm or adverse reactions
➤ A list of healthy foods that can minimize the risk of heart disease or cancer
➤ How to read food labels

Aside from the above, there are other essential information that offer additional choices to imbue a person with more consumer savvy, such as:

➤ A food guide pyramid one can adapt to one's taste and needs, which can be the basis for the grocery list
➤ A carbohydrate-protein ratio guide to incorporate in one's diet regimen
➤ A handy "food shopping guide" to bring to the supermarket will serve as a reminder on what foods to buy and what foods to avoid

All these and other helpful topics should help the reader wade through the maze of food hype and take control of one's eating lifestyle.

Let Food Be Your Medicine

~ Hippocrates

THE FOOD INDUSTRY

Chapter 1

The Food Jungle

Conflicting statements abound about what foods are "good" or "bad." Margarine was previously declared better than butter. Now, it seems that butter is the better alternative. If some food substances can cause harmful reactions, why is it still used in many products? Consumers are bombarded with advertising that has a lot of gimmicks that fall short of its promise, or are actually misleading. Theories on food combining, and the coming and going of new fad diets, add to the confusion of the shopper who just wants to eat a good and healthy meal.

Food shoppers today are not only interested in discounts or lower prices, they are also on the lookout for nutritional content in the foods they buy. Most shoppers now have been observed to take a long look at food labels printed in the packages. Shoppers know what foods they want. Do they know if these foods are good for their health? Everyone wants the best for their families. If they can obtain information about ingredients causing asthma, hives, toxicity or cancer, they would obviously not buy foods containing these substances.

You, the shopper, are in a dilemma. You do not have the time or the inclination to stand there amongst the food shelves in the supermarket, wondering and musing. Bringing a nutrition or reference book with you when you go shopping would be inconvenient and impractical. Not knowing what to do, you hurry from one shelf to the other, throwing caution to the wind. Then you buy whatever is cheaper, attractive, and offers a promised pleasure. You succumb to the easy way out.

In this modern age, fewer people prepare and cook their own foods. They prefer to eat out. They may buy fast foods, packaged, frozen, and ready-to-eat foods. This is an appropriate thing to do, now and then. However, done on a regular basis, one has actually placed his health and that of his family in the hands of an industry that has profit as its motive. To the health-conscious, it is time to take an interest in one's welfare. The consumer should not let others make up one's mind on what one should or should not eat. To be able to make informed choices on healthy eating, the consumer needs some important information on the following:

➤ Basic knowledge on safe and healthy eating
➤ How to gain access to relevant and new findings
➤ What are the agencies and who are the people involved in the food industry

The following pages should keep the food consumer on the right track, and, hopefully, help one to survive in the food jungle.

The Food Industry Today

The modernization of the food industry has done a lot of good to people living in the city. Modern food processing has made possible the availability of farm foods and foods from the sea, to cities and far-off places. Modern food preservation techniques such as canning, freezing, dehydrating, bottling, and other methods extend the shelf life of fresh foods. As a result, everyone has access to fruits, meat, dairy and vegetables, even several days or months after harvest or slaughter. Without proper processing techniques, food would suffer bacterial, mold, and fungal contamination. Foods would decompose, stink and look gross. This would cause serious illnesses and epidemics. The presence, therefore, of the food industry is much needed in modern societies. However, consumers are not hens in the poultry or milking cows in the dairy. They have a say on what they can consume and free to purchase a certain food or not. When consumers send a letter of praise or complaint to the manufacturer or agency concerned, they do the industry and themselves a favor. When a great number of consumers refuse to buy a certain product, the manufacturers know what that means. The food industry is not a one-way street.

Regulating the Food Industry

The food industry is regulated by several government agencies. The three prominent agencies are the U.S. Department of Agriculture (USDA), Food and Drug Administration (FDA), and the Environmental Protection Agency (EPA). There are private associations, institutions and consumer groups that also keep a watchful eye on the food industry. Some names of organizations and information sources can be found in Appendix A.

United States Department of Agriculture (USDA)

The USDA has a broad range of activities. It supports and promotes agriculture and the development of rural communities. It takes care of our forests, range lands, and food supply.

Food and Drug Administration (FDA)

The Pure Food Movement was started by Harvey H. Wiley, Chief of the Bureau of Chemistry in the U.S. Department of Agriculture. This resulted in the Pure Food and Drug Act, which restricted the use of harmful additives. It became a law despite objections and difficulties presented by food manufacturers and government officials. Twenty-five years later, the FDA was established. In 1938, the Food Drug and Cosmetic Act was passed. Several amendments came after this. It provided stronger measures to further consumer protection. The Food and Drug Administration is an operating division under the U.S. Department of Health and Human Services. It serves to protect the consumer by seeing to it that food is safe, pure and wholesome. The FDA also sees to it that animal drugs, medical devices, biological products, and electronic products are safe and effective.

Environmental Protection Agency (EPA)

The EPA is an independent agency that was established in December 2, 1970. Its duties are to minimize air and water pollution; and lessen health hazards and toxicity caused by pesticides, waste, and radiation. All pesticides are registered with EPA.

The Role of USDA, FDA, and EPA

The USDA, FDA, and the EPA are all federal agencies that take care of the environment and health of the citizenry. The EPA controls, regulates, and reduces the use of pesticide to ensure the safety of man, animals, and the environment. The FDA is responsible for the enforcement of regulations concerning the use of pesticides in food processing. The 1958 Food Additives Amendment banned the use of cancer-inducing additives and was known as a "zero-risk" policy. However, in 1989, EPA changed the "zero-risk" of exposing consumers to these kinds of additives to "negligible risk." This negligible risk policy allows the use of tolerable levels of pesticides in foods. With regards to our food supply, the USDA is responsible for the quality of our meat; the EPA, for our water needs; and the FDA, for the rest of our food supply.

For more information on certain regulations regarding the food industry, see Appendix A (Organization and Information Sources: Government).

FOOD ADDITIVES

Chapter 2

Food Additives

Food additives are chemicals or substances added to food to prevent it from spoiling. They add flavor, color, taste, attractive appearance, or nutrients. These substances will either change the characteristic of the food or become part of it. Additives are used in production, processing, transport, and food storage. They have more than 40 different uses. Salt, sugar, pepper, or vinegar are considered additives when added to food. Most additives can be seen or read in the list of ingredients in food packages.

Kinds of Food Additives

1. Classification as to whether it is added intentionally or not:

➤ Direct (intentional) – a substance added to food for a definite purpose. Example: aspartame added as a sweetener.
➤ Indirect (unintentional) – a molecule that becomes part of the food in trace amounts, as a result of its package, storage, or handling. Examples: plastic wrap molecules and lead from can solders.

2. Classification according to source:

➤ Natural substances – extracted from plants or other living things.
➤ Synthetic – a laboratory-made chemical to substitute for a natural substance.
➤ Wholly synthetic chemicals – these are also laboratory-made chemicals, but with no natural counterpart.

Whether an additive is natural or synthetic has no effect on the quality or safety of the chemical itself.

3. Classification according to usage:

➤ Preservatives – anti-microbial or antioxidant agents
➤ Texture – emulsifiers, stabilizers, thickeners
➤ Flavor enhancers
➤ Color
➤ Acid controllers
➤ Nutrients
➤ Bleaching and maturing agents
➤ Sweeteners
➤ Foaming agents or foaming inhibitors
➤ Clouding or clarifying agents
➤ Anti-caking or firming agents
➤ Sequestrants
➤ Humectants or drying agents
➤ Leavenings

Regulating Additive Use

Additives have been used since ancient times. Today, there are almost 3,000 additives used in modern food processing. The Food Amendment Act of 1958 stipulates that manufacturers have to prove that the use of an additive in a product is safe. FDA needs to approve this safety factor before it can be used. Exempted from these provisions are the following:

1. Prior-sanctioned substances – These are additives that were determined by FDA or the Department of Agriculture, as safe, prior to the Food Amendment Act of 1958. Examples are sodium nitrite and potassium nitrite.
2. Generally Recognized as Safe (GRAS) – These are additives used before 1958 and recognized by experts as safe, based on its history of use or on published scientific evidence. Examples are sugar, salt, and monosodium glutamate.

If new evidence proves that a prior sanctioned or GRAS substance is not safe, the additive will either be banned for use or re-evaluated. It takes a long time to remove an additive from the market. This is due to data collection and time-consuming hearings. New additives also take a few years before it can be used. Many tests need to be done before introducing it to the market.

"Absolute" and "Reasonable" Certainty

The FDA has done numerous evaluations of tests and research results on food additives. Great strides have been made in trying to give consumers safe and healthy foods. This is a far cry from the conditions in the 19th century when food supply was contaminated, adulterated, and mislabeled rampantly. This does not mean to say that all foods in the market are fully guaranteed to be completely safe for the general public.

Every year, several new additives are being recommended to the FDA for approval. Scientific knowledge constantly evolves based on new findings. Decisions about food safety are based on scientific evidence available at that time. "Absolute certainty" about additives cannot be proven. There is only "reasonable certainty" that using it will cause no harm. This judgement is based on average individual use. It does not take into consideration special populations with ailments or specific sensitivities. Some substances are allowed even though it may be harmful to a few people or animals. To protect the consumer, a margin of safety at the level of 1/100th of the harmful amount is set as the limit.

Because of myriad differences in our physiological make up, one man's food may be another man's poison. For this reason, consumers should check out food labels. This is especially necessary if you have diabetes, heart disease, high blood pressure, severe allergies, phenylketonuria, or other ailments. It also matters if you are buying food for a child or a pregnant woman. When adverse reactions to food occur, you can report this to the FDA so they are aware of the matter. Sometimes, the consumers fail to inform the FDA. Thus, this agency may not be able to respond accordingly.

Food Additives That Can Cause Harm Or Adverse Reactions

An appropriate consumer response to food additives that can cause harm or adverse reactions is to avoid them altogether.

Avoid

➤ Acesulfame K or Acesulfame Potassium, Sweet One, Sunette
➤ Aspartame or NutraSweet, NatraTaste, Equal, Sweet Thing, Fifty 50, Spoonful
➤ Cyclamate
➤ Saccharin or Sweet 'N Low, Sweet 10, Sugar Twin
➤ Nitrites or Nitrates
➤ Sulfites or Sulphites
➤ Potassium Bromate
➤ Brominated Vegetable Oil (BVO)
➤ Irradiated Foods
➤ Recombinant Bovine Growth Hormone (rBGH) or Recombinant Bovine Somatotropin (rBST)
➤ Hydrogenated Vegetable Oil, or Hardened Oil, or Partially Hydrogenated Oil
➤ MSG (Monosodium Glutamate)
➤ HVP (Hydrolyzed Vegetable Protein or Autolyzed Yeast)
➤ BHA (Butylated Hydroxyanisole)
➤ BHT (Butylated Hydroxytoluene)
➤ TBHQ (Tertiary Butylhydroquinone)
➤ Aluminum compounds
➤ Quinine
➤ Olestra
➤ Citrus Red No. 2

➤ FD & C Red No. 3 (Erythrosine)

➤ FD & C Blue No.1 (Brilliant Blue)

➤ FD & C Blue No. 2 (Indigotine or Indigo Carmine)

➤ FD & C Green No. 3 (Fast Green)

➤ FD & C Yellow No. 6 (Sunset Yellow)

➤ FD & C Red No. 40 (Allura AC)

➤ FD & C Yellow No. 5 (Tartrazine)

➤ Cochineal (Carminic Acid, or Carmine of Cochineal)

The additives to avoid are known to combine two or more of the following characteristics:

➤ Suspected or proven to cause cancer

➤ Causes life-threatening or highly adverse reactions

➤ Highly controversial

➤ Too many consumer complaints against it

➤ Existing contradictory claims requiring further testing

➤ Available in minute amounts as an ingredient, but present in foods consumed in significantly large quantity on a regular basis

Know More About Additives

The information in the following pages is based on current research results and studies at the time of writing. Research results and studies sometimes contradict each other or are open to conflicting interpretations. These additives are the more common ones, and should others become known to you, just add it to your "avoid" list. It is not possible to come up with a static list, because new complaints and discoveries will always crop up. This list may grow with time, and then, some additives may be removed from the list if the food manufacturers no longer use them. The purpose of this list is to make the consumer aware of the hidden dangers in foods. It is hoped that this will motivate the consumer to be vigilant and take initiative to learn and find out more about the food one normally eats. The reader may draw his own conclusions and, hopefully, choose to err on the side of caution.

The food colors mentioned above have a more profound effect on children and can affect their behavior and mental status, aside from other allergic reactions. Food colors do not provide nutrients and do not affect the flavor of the food. See page 51 about food allergy and other reactions.

Artificial Sweeteners

Acesulfame K (acesulfame potassium) – This sweetener is sold to food manufacturers under the name of Sunette or Sweet One. It is an artificial high-intensity sweetener that is 200 times sweeter than table sugar. It is composed of carbon, nitrogen, oxygen, hydrogen, sulfur, and potassium atoms. It is non-caloric and sodium-free. The body does not metabolize acesulfame. When used in large quantities, it loses its clean sweet taste. It can be used in cooking and does not affect blood glucose levels.

The manufacturer's numerous tests done in the 1970's were evaluated by FDA. Some health professionals saw some flaws and inadequacies in the tests, which did not negate the carcinogenicity of the sweetener. It is believed to cause cancer in animals. In 1988, FDA approved its use only in dry beverages and dessert mixes, candies, lozenges, and chewing gum. In July 1998, approval was finally given, allowing acesulfame K to be used also in diet soda drinks.

Aspartame – It is sold under the brand names NutraSweet, Equal, Natrataste, Sweet Thing, Fifty 50, and Spoonful. It is 200 times sweeter than table sugar. High temperatures in cooking will cause it to lose its sweetness. It is present in various foods and drugs today that are considered "sugar-free." Aspartame is made up of two amino acids, phenylalanine and aspartic acid, held in chemical bond by methanol (also known as wood alcohol). Dissenters to the use of aspartame maintain that when aspartame breaks down in the bloodstream, methanol toxicity is a possibility. Side effects include headaches, blurred vision, stomach pains, depression and nausea. Although methanol is present in a lot of natural foods, it has other components, especially ethyl alcohol, which neutralizes the harmful effect of methanol. Aspartame breaks down into phenylalanine, aspartic acid and methanol, but has no ethyl alcohol. If liquid beverages, like diet soda drinks, are exposed to temperatures over 85°F during summer season, chemical decomposition can occur and freestanding methanol exists in the product. The FDA and manufacturers of this sweetener maintain that methanol (as a breakdown of aspartame) in the body is harmless because it is in very small amounts. Compared to other natural foods it does not accumulate in the body to reach harmful levels.

Discovered in 1965, the FDA approved its use in 1974. However, this sweetener was prevented from being sold, as a result of protests from consumer groups. This led to studies made by a panel of pathologists appointed by the FDA. The FDA gave the clearance in 1981 for its use as tabletop sweetener and dry beverage mix. In 1983, it was approved for use in carbonated drinks like diet sodas. Later, the FDA extended its use as an "inactive ingredient" in pharmaceutical use and as an additive for all other foods for which it had no previous approval. Like the other sweeteners before it, aspartame is widely used by several countries and found safe by the JECFA (Joint Committee on Food Additives) of the UN-FAO and WHO.

After the conduct of some researches, it was alleged at some point in time that aspartame causes bladder and brain tumors. The FDA, however, claimed that research reviews indicated the safety of the additive. Nonetheless, about 3,000 complaints (and more trickling in) were received by the FDA against the use of aspartame. The FDA believed that these are mild complaints in normal living, and they should be directed to their physician. Most complaints result from the use of diet sodas and table sweeteners.

A small portion of the population suffers from a rare disease called Phenylketonuria. These individuals lack an enzyme to process phenylalanine. This deficiency will result in the accumulation of phenylalanine in the blood causing brain damage and mental retardation. There are about 15,000 in the USA and millions of Americans may be carriers of PKU genes, although they are not phenylketonuric themselves. Products containing aspartame must, therefore, carry a warning on the label that says: "Phenylketonurics: contains Phenylalanine."

Cyclamate – Cyclamate is made up of either sodium cyclamate or calcium cyclamate. It is only 30 times sweeter than table sugar and, therefore, has the least sweetening power compared to the other artificial sweeteners. It is stable in hot and cold temperatures and soluble in liquids.

A previous experiment showing a result of bladder tumors in rats led to the banning of cyclamate in the USA in 1970. The FDA and manufacturers criticized the test. There were lots of controversies that arose, and due to pressure from consumer groups and Congress, cyclamate was finally banned. In 1985, the FDA reviewed the cyclamate case and declared that it did not cause cancer, after all. Some consumer groups still believe it can cause cancer. It is currently being used in Europe and other countries. The manufacturers of cyclamate are trying to push for its comeback in the USA.

Saccharin – Saccharin is a non-caloric petroleum derivative, which is 300 times sweeter than table sugar. It comes under the brand names Sweet 'N Low, Sweet 10, and Sugar Twin. Saccharin is not metabolized by the human body and has no effect on blood sugar. It has a bitter after-taste, specially after heating. Developed in 1879, it was used as a food preservative and antiseptic. Saccharin has been used for more than a hundred years. It is used in a variety of processed foods such as soft drinks, baked goods, chewing gum, candies, desserts, and salad dressings. Findings in several tests done in the United States showed bladder tumor in rats. Canadian tests also showed bladder cancer. During the 1970's, saccharin was the only non-caloric sweetener used in the USA. In 1972, after several studies, the FDA restricted its use only as a tabletop sweetener. In

1977, U.S. Congress passed the "Saccharin Study and Labeling Act" to stop the FDA restriction. This moratorium on the saccharin ban has been extended six times. The last moratorium, as of this writing will expire on May 1, 2002. However, in 1991, the FDA formally withdrew its saccharin ban. Diet drinks and tabletop sweeteners are required to bear this label, stating:

"Use of this product may be hazardous to your health. This product contains saccharin, which has been determined to cause cancer in laboratory animals."

Last December 1998, the National Toxicology Program recommended dropping saccharin from its cancer-causing list. A non-profit health advocacy group called the Center for Science in the Public Interest (CSPI) has voiced its objection to the de-listing of saccharin because of uncertainty that still exists. Great Britain puts severe restriction in its use, while it is available only by prescription in France.

New Artificial Sweeteners

Sucralose – Sucralose is made from sugar, tastes like sucrose, but is not recognized by the body as sugar or carbohydrates. This artificial sweetener is made through a process whereby three chlorine atoms are substituted for three hydrogen-oxygen groups belonging to the sugar molecule. Sucralose touts many benefits such as clean taste with no aftertaste, highly stable in hot or cold temperatures, does not affect blood sugar, does not accumulate in the body, and is non-caloric. It is 600 times sweeter than table sugar. In April 1998, the FDA approved the use of sucralose in beverages, desserts, and in a variety of food products, after 100 thorough scientific tests over a 20-year period. It will be marketed under the brand name of Splenda. It is being used in 29 countries including Australia, Canada and South America. This sweetener seems to be highly favored over the other artificial sweeteners by concerned consumer groups.

Alitame – Alitame is another non-caloric artificial sweetener that awaits FDA approval. It is 2,000 times sweeter than table sugar and is made up of amino acids, L-aspartic acid and D-alanine and a novel amine. It has a clean taste and remains stable at high temperatures, except in some acidic solutions requiring long storage. Its uses are similar to the other sweeteners. Animal and human studies have been made with regard to food safety. Presently, alitame has been approved for use in Australia, New Zealand, Mexico and the Peoples Republic of China. Its brand name is Aclame.

Is There A Future For Artificial Sweeteners?

After this book goes into print, we may still hear of other new artificial sweeteners being introduced into the market. Manufacturers sometimes combine sweeteners so that each one may offset deficiencies in the other. The combination can serve to improve flavor, increase stability, and lower processing costs. Examples are combination of cyclamate with saccharin and acesulfame K with aspartame. Artificial sweeteners are supposed to be a boon to diabetics and the obese. This should mean that there is less consumption of table sugar or sucrose. Instead, Americans are still using a lot of refined sugars.

Natural Alternative Sweeteners

Stevia – This is a plant belonging to the Compositae family. Its scientific name is *Stevia rebandiana bertoni* and is native to South America. Today, it is grown in several countries. It is 200 times sweeter than table sugar. For centuries, the Guarani Indians have been using the leaves of this plant as a sweetener for their tea, and also for other medicinal purposes. Now, Stevia is planted here in the USA, Canada, and Europe.

Since 1970, Japan has been the largest consumer of stevioside. In 1996, stevioside cornered 41% of the sweetener products in Japan. In 1994, the FDA removed its import ban on Stevia on the condition that it be marked as a "dietary supplement" and not as a sweetener. Proponents for Stevia consider it non-caloric, does not affect blood sugar, is heat stable to 392°F (200°C) and non-toxic.

➤ **Blackstrap molasses** – contains calcium, iron, potassium, thiamin, riboflavin, niacin, B-6, phosphorus, and copper

➤ **Brown Sugar** – contains calcium, magnesium, and iron

➤ **Honey** – contains Vitamin C, thiamin, riboflavin, niacin, calcium, phosphorus, and copper

Nitrates and Nitrites

Nitrates and nitrites come in different names, such as sodium or potassium nitrite, and sodium or potassium nitrate.

Nitrites have been around as food preservatives for over 2,000 years. Presently, these are used for curing meat products such as bacon, hot dogs, ham, corned beef, deli meats, luncheon meats, and smoked fish. Aside from preserving meat, it adds a brighter red color to meat. Bratwursts, which do not contain nitrites, are pale in color. Nitrites retard the growth of bacteria (*Clostridium botulinum*) that causes botulism poisoning, and retain the attractive color of fresh meat.

In itself, nitrates and nitrites do not cause cancer. Nitrates readily turn into nitrites while in the stomach. Nitrites combine with chemical compounds called secondary or tertiary amines (derivatives of ammonia) that occurs naturally in food. The nitrites react with amines to form nitrosamines, which can cause a variety of cancers. This reaction occurs before cooking (in the shelf or in the refrigerator), during cooking (at 370°F or higher), and in the digestive system of animals or human, when ingested.

Nitrites belong to the "Prior-Sanctioned Substances" category, since they were already used before the Food Additives Amendment Act of 1958. As a result of studies made, the government has reduced the use of nitrites in food. Natural nitrates occur in vegetables while natural nitrites occur in our saliva. In the case of vegetables, its built-in nutrients and fiber inhibit the formation of nitrosamines. Cured meats are usually poor sources of protein, plus, they are high in fat and sodium. These contain amines and concentrated doses of nitrites. In Canada, use of nitrites in fish or fish products is banned.

Alternatives to Meat Products Containing Nitrites

There are a number of meat products that may not contain nitrites, namely:

➤ Bratwurst
➤ Frozen meat products that state "uncured"
➤ Fresh meat
➤ Uncured cooked sausages
➤ Uncured frankfurters
➤ Uncured bacon
➤ Pork bellies
➤ Pork strips

Some food processors of meat products containing nitrites, add Vitamin E or Vitamin C to block nitrosamine formation. If you must buy cured meats with nitrites, check the label for the presence of these two vitamins. They may also add different versions of these vitamins, under the following names:

➤ Ascorbate acid
➤ Ascorbic acid
➤ Sodium ascorbate
➤ Potassium ascorbate
➤ Erythorbic acid
➤ Ascorbyl palmitate
➤ Tocopherols

Upon purchase, meat products (without nitrite treatment) must be cooked or frozen immediately, in order to limit their exposure to bacterial contamination.

Sulfites

Sulfites or sulfur-based preservatives are also known in food labels as sulfur dioxide; sodium or potassium sulfite; sodium or potassium bisulfite and sodium or potassium metabisulfite. Sulfites have been used around the world for centuries. Its first known use was as a preservative in wine. It is still used today in beer and wine, potato products, cider juices, soft drinks, and dried fruits to prevent growth of bacteria during fermentation. Its other uses include the following:

➤ Prevent oxidation or the discoloration of fruits and vegetables
➤ Prevent melanosis or dark pigmentation on shrimps and lobsters
➤ Condition dough
➤ Bleach food starches
➤ Maintain stability and potency of some pharmaceuticals

About one million Americans are considered sensitive to sulfites. Hundreds of complaints have been lodged with the FDA, ranging from mild to life threatening cases. Asthma sufferers are more prone to sulfite sensitivity. Some complaints are: difficulty in breathing, hives, vomiting, diarrhea, abdominal cramps and pain, swelling of the tongue, and loss of consciousness. As a result of these complaints, the FDA has taken the following actions:

➤ Banned the use of sulfites on fresh vegetables and fruits in salad bars where these are expected to be eaten raw.
➤ Ordered listing of sulfites in cooked, packaged, and processed foods on labels if they are more than 10 ppm (parts per million). Aside from this, its function in the food has also to be stated.

As a result of FDA measures, complaints involving sulfites have decreased. However, consumers need to avoid or limit their intake, depending on the severity of a person's sensitivity to sulfites. Individuals allergic or sensitive to sulfites should read food labels in order to avoid using food products containing this additive. Excessive amounts of sulfites in the body can rob one of Vitamin B-1 (thiamine).

Potassium Bromate

Potassium bromate is used as an oxidizer in breads and other flour products to improve volume, texture, and baking performance. Bromate breaks down to bromide during fermentation and baking. The question is, "how much bromate is really left after baking?" One side of the controversy believes that the breakdown is not complete. The other side, on the basis of some data, assumes that there are no bromate residues if potassium bromate is lowered to 15-30 ppm, coupled with the use of ferrous sulfate, bleached flour, and ascorbic acid – plus increasing fermentation time, baking temperature, and baking time. Some side effects of this additive are nausea, vomiting, diarrhea, and pain. It is considered as a mutagen that has the potential to cause cancer in animal tests. In 1991, the FDA requested the food industry to reduce the usage levels of potassium bromide. At this time, it is not known whether action has been taken or if any action taken was appropriate. Potassium bromate is banned in California, Canada, Japan and most European countries.

Alternatives to Potassium Bromate

Consumers will not know if certain bread contains potassium bromate. It will not be listed in the label. Most bread makers who do not use it will state if their bread has "no bromate," or if it is "unbromated," or "bromate-free." Examples of these found in our local groceries are "Pepperidge Farm" and "Nature's Own." There may be other unbromated brands that we are not aware of at this time.

Brominated Vegetable Oil (BVO)

BVO is a mixture of bromine liquid and vegetable oil. It is used as an additive in some soda drinks and processed juices. Vegetable oils used can either be corn, cottonseed, olive, or sesame oil. When BVO is used, the oil and liquid does not separate, giving the liquid a cloudy appearance or an illusion of a fresh natural juice. Traces of BVO accumulate in the body tissues causing biological changes. One of them is the reduction of histamines in the body. Thus, making it difficult to fight allergies and infection. A study in Canada showed heart, liver, thyroid and kidney damage to rats given feeds with BVO for eighty days. The FDA has removed it from the GRAS list, but it is still legal for manufacturers to use it. Meanwhile, the FDA has imposed severe limitation on the amount used until completion of further studies. Consumer groups are demanding more tests and re-evaluation of this substance.

Alternatives to BVO

Instead of drinking soda drinks or other juices with BVO, go for the real thing. Eat fresh fruits, or drink freshly squeezed juice, or natural juice drinks without any artificial color or flavor additive.

Food Irradiation

Food irradiation or *cold pasteurization* is exposing foods to radioactive isotopes (radioisotopes) in varying doses, depending on the type of product. The purpose of radiation is sterilization and preservation, thus, giving the product a longer shelf life. Radioisotopes used are either Cobalt 60 or Caesium 137. Cobalt 60 is manufactured while Caesium 137 is a by-product of nuclear weaponry. Presently, only Cobalt 60 is being used. When the limited supply runs out, Caesium 137 will be used.

The irradiation process takes place in a room specially built for this purpose. An irradiation room would have concrete walls 6 to 8 feet thick. Food in conveyor belts would move on top of a pool of water containing radioactive rods, which rise up to bombard the food with gamma rays. The dosage is in terms of "rads" (Roentgen absorbed dose) or "kilograys," which differs according to the type of food.

Thirty-nine (39) countries permit food irradiation or "cold pasteurization," but only 29 are presently using it. In the USA, the FDA approved the irradiation of beef and lamb, last December 1997. Poultry, fruits, vegetables, pork and grains had been given irradiation permits previous to this date on different occasions. Herbs and spices are now being irradiated in the USA.

Contrary to some common notions, irradiated food does not become radioactive, unless there are radiation leaks, human error, or equipment malfunctioning. Irradiation helps control the two chief causes of food-borne illness – *Salmonella* and *Campylobacter*. This process kills insects, parasites, *E. coli* bacteria, 90% of the microorganisms, and delays ripening and sprouting. On the other hand, this is an expensive technology that is not totally effective against viruses and other organisms, when used in recommended doses. This process would not totally destroy *Clostridium botulinum,* which causes food poisoning. Vitamin levels can be reduced in irradiation and reduced even further in the cooking process. Some vitamin losses are in Vitamins A, E, C, K, and B-1. Irradiation creates new chemical compounds in treated foods called unique radiolytic products (URPs) or (RPs). These still need to be studied to find out if they are carcinogenic or mutagenic. Irradiation causes change in certain foods in terms of color and flavor. It may destroy food enzymes, which aid in digestion.

In the international scene, proponents are: the United Nations International Atomic Energy (IAEA), the Food and Agriculture Organization (FAO), and the World Health Organization (WHO).

In the USA, those favoring the use of radiation are the Department of Energy (DOE), the U.S. Department of Agriculture (USDA), the FDA, the National Safety Database, the American Dietetic Association, the National Pork Producers Council, and some food manufacturers.

On the other side are some concerned consumer groups and experts. They state that tests done in different countries showed some harmful effects, such as: tumors, kidney ailment, testicular damage, mutations, and reduced fertility, to name a few. Those who favor irradiation contend that it is safe for the consumer and that the RP's are composed of naturally occurring chemicals in foods. Granting that irradiated food is totally safe, there are still fears about radioactive discharge in the environment. If more facilities for irradiation are set up, there will be more chances of accidents inside facilities; or in the transporting of the isotopes, in case of traffic accidents.

The DOE plans to build food irradiation facilities in Hawaii, Alaska, Washington, and Florida. In 1998, Hawaii residents have already voiced their objections to the setting up of an irradiation facility in their State. Canada provides 90% of the world supply of cobalt 60, although no irradiated food is being sold locally in its market place. This is due to the presence of vigilant consumer groups in Canada. These consumer groups are presently fighting for the phase-out of nuclear power by proposing the use of safer energy sources substitutes. Countries banning food irradiation are New Zealand, Austria, Germany, Romania, Switzerland, U.K., Sweden, Abu Dhabi, The Dominican Republic, Botswana, Ethiopia, Kenya, and Tanzania.

Food irradiation falls under the description of "additives." In this context, it falls under the FDA rules and restrictions. Advocates of food irradiation claim that it is not an additive, but a "process." If it is a process, restrictions and further studies on irradiation can be reduced. The FDA, however, has made it known that whether it is a "process" or an "additive," irradiation will still require the same restrictions as additives. In the USA, New York and Maine have banned the sale of irradiated foods. New York exempts spices from the ban.

Dealing With Irradiation

Does one know if a food has been irradiated? Not always. Labels on frozen potato by-products, spices, and irradiated potatoes in some canned soup will not list irradiation as an ingredient. As for the rest of the food supply, you have to look for the irradiation symbol in the food package. This symbol is called the "radura," which is shown below:

RADURA

To a person who is not familiar with the radura symbol, the plant-like figure will seem to falsely represent something organic or coming from nature. If you are concerned about irradiation, familiarize yourself with the radura symbol, in case the following warning is not stated in the package.

"Treated with Radiation," "Irradiated,"
or "Treated with ionizing radiation."

McCormick Company has declared that it does not irradiate their spices and will state it in the spice labels should they do so.

Recombinant Bovine Growth Hormone (rBGH)

This hormone is also known as Recombinant Bovine Somatotropin (rBST). It is a genetically engineered growth hormone that can increase milk production in cows from 10 to 25 percent. The use of BGH increases the amount of the protein hormone – Insulin-like Growth Factor-One (IGF-1) in cow's milk.

The regular use of this hormone leads to increased mastitis in cows. Mastitis is an inflammation of the breast or udder of the cow as a result of infection. This leads to frequent use of antibiotics, among cows treated with BGH, which would end up in the consumer's milk. One study showed that BGH milk had increased fat and less casein (milk protein) content. This is also believed to cause tumors in the colon, breast, and prostate.

FDA approved the use of BGH in 1994, and is marketed under the brand name "Posilac." Presently, we have an oversupply of milk which makes the small dairy farmer not too happy with this product. Pushing the supply to excess will lead to a drop in prices, which will force the small farmers out of business. In December 1994, the Commission of the European Community placed a moratorium on the use of BGH until the year 2000. Twelve countries are presently using BGH.

Alternatives to BGH/BST Treated Milk and Milk Products

The FDA does not require food products to be labeled when "BGH-free." Labeling is voluntary as long as assertions are truthful and not misleading. Unfortunately, some States have policies or laws forbidding the declaration of "BGH-free" on food labels. It is, therefore, difficult to ascertain on milk products coming from these States, if it is BGH-free or not. If the presence of BGH on milk does not bother you, then you do not have a problem. If it is a cause for concern, the safe route is to read labels. Some producers have statements on their labels saying that:

"Our farms produced this milk without the use of hormones, antibiotics, or pesticides"

or

"BGH/BST-free"

Even when buying organic dairy, it is still a good idea to read the labels. A list of some "BGH-free" dairy producers is found in Appendix B, pages 222-223.

Hydrogenated Vegetable Oil

Hydrogenated vegetable oil is also known as "hardened oil," "vegetable fat," or "partially hydrogenated oil." Hydrogenation is the process of subjecting polyunsaturated vegetable oil to high heat and great pressure. Hydrogen atoms are caused to be added to the oil. The end result is the transformation of liquid oil to a semi-solid state. This makes the product spreadable, such as margarine. For commercial purposes, the oil needs to be firmed up. Otherwise, the consumer will be pouring the oil on the bread. For longer storage, hydrogenation prevents the oil from turning rancid. Before the vegetable oil is hydrogenated, it contains essential fatty acids, which are needed by the body to promote and maintain good health. When exposed to high heat, these fatty acids are converted to polymers, which are similar to varnish, shellac, and plastics. This chemical change transforms the essential fatty acids into trans fatty acids. These trans fatty acids are officially typecast as unsaturated fats, but they act like saturated fats. Trans fatty acids resulting from hydrogenation are deposited in different amounts in body tissues. These affect the normal function of organs. In animal studies, this effect on organs resulted in susceptibility to cancer, gallstone formation, lower levels of good cholesterol, and growth retardation. It also causes skin, hair and nail problems, and weakened blood sugar metabolism. Other studies indicate, though, that it does lesser harms than saturated fats, in terms of blood cholesterol levels, only. Hydrogenated vegetable oil can be found in some snack foods like potato chips, peanut butter, frozen foods, margarine, cakes, and pastries.

Dealing with Hydrogenated Vegetable Oils:

➤ Read the labels.
➤ If you must use margarine, select the softer one. Use sparingly, as you also should, with butter.

Monosodium Glutamate (MSG)

MSG is a "free glutamate" released by the breakdown of glutamic acid. It comes in the form of a crystalline substance like salt and sugar. It enhances flavor by stimulating the taste buds. Ajinomoto, Vetsin, and Accent are some of its brand names. Some adverse reactions have been noted after eating foods containing MSG, such as the following:

➤ Burning sensation, numbness or tingling in the back of the neck
➤ Tightness or pain in the chest
➤ Headaches
➤ Nausea
➤ Rapid heartbeat
➤ Difficulty in breathing
➤ Drowsiness and weakness
➤ Skin rash

Almost all of the above symptoms are transitory and do not present serious medical problems. In addition, this sensitivity does not happen to all that ingest MSG. It is theorized that people deficient in Vitamin B-6 (Pyridoxine) are more prone to this reaction. This type of individuals may not include MSG in their food until they overcome this deficiency. In 1970, MSG was linked to brain damage in laboratory animal infants. The manufacturers, then, consented to stop adding MSG to baby food. However, glutamates do exist naturally in the human body and in common foods like bouillon, tomatoes, and cheese. Commercially, it is used as an additive in broth, soups, processed condiments, fried chicken batter, salad dressing, processed meat and some potato chips. Other additives that contain glutamates are as follows:

➤ Hydrolyzed vegetable protein (HVP)
➤ Hydrolyzed plant protein
➤ Hydrolyzed protein

➤ Calcium caseinate
➤ Sodium caseinate
➤ Texturized protein
➤ Autolyzed yeast
➤ Yeast extract
➤ Hydrolyzed oat flour

Dealing with MSG/HVP:

➤ Look at food labels and minimize the use of foods containing MSG.
➤ If you are sensitive to MSG, request to omit it in your food order when dining out in restaurants.

BHA, BHT, and TBHQ

➤ BHA – Butylated Hydroxyanisole
➤ BHT – Butylated Hydroxytoluene
➤ TBHQ – Tertiary butylhydroquinone

BHA, BHT, and TBHQ are often used together. They are petroleum-based antioxidants designed to prevent the product from turning rancid, or from losing its flavor or color. They are sometimes sprayed on the insides of cereal or cheese packages.

TBHQ is believed to be toxic in very low doses. Like BHA and BHT, it affects behavior, especially in children, as related to sleep patterns, aggression, and weight loss. They cause rashes and have been linked to cancer in animals. They are used as additives in a lot of snack foods that children eat. Some of them are Jell-O, potato chips, cereals, candies, gums, and pork sausages. BHT is banned as a food additive in England. On the other hand, other studies showed that BHA and BHT blocked the action of chemical carcinogens that could cause stomach cancer. They also believe that these preservatives prevent the breakdown of Vitamin A and D.

Dealing with BHA, BHT and TBHQ:

In view of the contradictory claims, the safer way is to minimize use of products containing these additives, until it is ascertained to be actually safe for children.

Aluminum Compounds

Aluminum is found in a wide range of products from food to electrical transmission lines and auto radiators, to mention a few. As a food additive, it is used for firming, anti-caking, defoaming, and as a carrier for bleaching. It comes under the following names:

➤ Aluminum ammonium sulfate
➤ Aluminum calcium sulfate
➤ Aluminum chloride
➤ Aluminum stearate
➤ Aluminum sulfate
➤ Aluminum potassium sulfate
➤ Sodium aluminum
➤ Sodium aluminum phosphate or aluminum baking powder
➤ Sodium aluminum silicate or sodium silicaaluminate
➤ Sodium aluminum sulfate

These are found in baking powders, pickles, cheese, pancakes and waffle mixes, and in chewing gums. Aside from food products, aluminum can steal into our system in small amounts through our drinking water, some household products, deodorants, and antacids.

Aluminum is metabolized systemically by the body. The kidneys and the digestive system dispose off some of it. The amount the body absorbs depends on what nutrients are present at the time of ingestion:

➤ Nutrients that inhibit the absorption of aluminum are calcium, zinc, phosphorus and fluorine.
➤ Nutrients that intensify absorption of aluminum are iron, Vitamin D, and citrates.

It seems that there is more aluminum absorption among older persons. Aluminum is a selective neurotoxin. When absorbed in the bloodstream, it exhibits affinity for the brain. Aluminum treated water was previously used in dialysis patients. It built up in their bodies to toxic levels which led to "dialysis dementia" – a fatal neurological disease. Dialysis patients now use aluminum-free water in their artificial kidneys. Alzheimer's disease is suspected to be caused by aluminum in the brain. However, research conducted by the Alzheimer's Disease and Related Disorders Association (ARDA) found no connection between aluminum and this disease.

Dealing with Aluminum:

➤ Buy baking powder containing sodium tartrate.
➤ Aluminum in drinking water can be removed by "reverse osmosis."
➤ If concerned with aluminum in the diet, check out the ingredients in the food labels.

Quinine

Quinine or quinine sulfate is an alkaloid obtained from the cinchona tree found mostly in the tropics. It is derived from the bark of its trunks, branches, and roots. It is mainly used to treat malaria caused by *Plasmodium falciparum*. A secondary use is for the treatment of night muscle cramps. As a food additive, it is used in soda drinks, like quinine water or bitter lemon. This additive is poorly tested. Side effects from regular and high doses are not established. For individuals sensitive to quinine, small doses can lead to skin rashes, itching, and possibly asthma. Since it is a muscle relaxant, it should be avoided by patients with *Myasthenia gravis*. Pregnant women should avoid drinks containing quinine. It is suspected that quinine can cause birth defects.

Dealing with Quinine:

➤ Read labels on soda drinks if you want to avoid this additive.

➤ Buy organic or fresh fruit juice drinks as alternative beverages.

Olestra

Olestra or "sucrose polyester" is a synthetic fat substitute. After several researches done by the manufacturer, the FDA approved the use of Olestra in 1996, under the brand name "Olean." This no-calorie fat additive is indigestible and passes unchanged through the digestive system. It can take the heat of deep-frying without chemical breakdown. Health experts are afraid that, since products containing Olestra are fat free, consumers will increase their intake, forgetting that the product still contains calories. Products that contain Olestra are mostly potato chips. Unpleasant effects resulting from eating foods with Olestra occur in some people. These people experience digestive problems such as stomach cramping, diarrhea, fecal urgency, nausea, and flatulence. Heavy consumers of these foods may also have unwanted "anal leakage" which can leave oil residues in the toilet or cause underwear staining.

Another cause for concern is that Olestra absorbs the fat soluble vitamins. These are vitamins A, D, E and K. This deprives the body of the benefits of these nutrients. Studies also showed that it could lower the levels of carotenoids, alphacarotene, beta carotene, lutein, and lycopene, which help protect eyesight.

Dealing with Olestra:

Since Olestra (Olean) is a new additive in the market, you need to go easy in consuming the product that lists it as an ingredient. The food product will contain the following statements:

"This product contains Olestra. Olestra may cause abnormal cramping and loose stools. Olestra inhibits the absorption of some vitamins and other nutrients. Vitamins A, D, E, and K have been added."

Children, old people and pregnant women should especially exercise caution in eating snack foods with Olestra or use other low fat foods as an alternative.

Food Colors

Colors are used in foods, drugs, and cosmetics. Food color additives are listed as "FD & C" which means they can be used in food, drugs and cosmetics. "D & C" means they can be used only in drugs and cosmetics. Color additives are either:

➤ Certifiable (certified) – These additives are man-made and have to undergo some tests to gain approval from the FDA; or

➤ Exempt from certification (non-certified) – These come from natural sources or are man-made replicas of a product of nature. They can be derived from plant, animals, organisms, and minerals.

An example of a certified food color is FD & C RED No. 3; and an example of a non-certified food color is turmeric. Certified color additives are used as "dyes" or "lakes." "Dyes" dissolve in water and are used in candies, beverages, baked goods, dairy products, and pet foods. "Lakes" are not water-soluble and are used in products containing fats and oils. "Lakes" are also used in products where "bleeding" or leaching of color would mess up the appearance of a product. These are found in cookies, fillings, chewing gums, doughnut mixes, and candies.

The use of synthetic color additives in food is more aesthetic than essential, because it has nothing to do with the nutritive value of the food. These colors are used to make the food more attractive, to have uniformity in color and to provide food identification, such as red for cherry. With the passage of the Pure Food and Drug Acts of 1906, the FDA started to make an assessment of color additives. As a result, a lot of harmful color additives were banned. The different food colors used presently are the following:

Common Names	Other Names	Hue
Citrus Red No2	None	Orange
FD&C Red No3	Erythrosine	Cherry Red
FD&C Blue No1	Brilliant Blue	Bright Blue
FD&C Blue No2	Indigotine	Royal Blue
FD&C Green No3	Fast Green	Sea Green
FD&C Yellow No6	Sunset Yellow	Orange Yellow
FD&C Yellow No5	Tartrazine	Lemon Yellow
FD&D Red No40	Allura Red AC	Orange Red
Cochineal	Carminic Acid	Bright Red

Avoid these Food Colors:

Citrus Red No. 2 – It is used to color the skin of pale oranges to give it the right shade identified with the fruit and to give the oranges a uniform color. Studies in mice with regard to the use of this color showed cancer and chromosomal damages. It is believed that this additive does not seep through the orange peel, and the inner fruit is safe. Avoid using the skin for cooking, unless you are sure that it is free from Citrus Red. No. 2.

FD & C Red No. 3 (Erythrosine) – The FDA banned the use of this color in 1990. It was shown to cause thyroid tumor in rats. It also affects human behavior and moods. The ban affects cosmetics but not foods. The administration at that time overruled the FDA and allowed its use "until supplies are used up." At present, there is no indication as to when the supplies will be used up. It is used mostly on cherries in fruit cocktail, in candies, and baked products.

FD & C Blue No. 1 (Brilliant Blue) - It is found in desserts, confectioneries, candies, and beverages. It has not been properly tested and suspected to contain a small cancer risk. It is banned in Finland and France.

FD & C Blue No. 2 (Indigotine/Indigo-carmine) – Not much is known of this additive, although, it was suspected to cause brain tumors in animals. It can cause allergic reactions. Aside from soft drinks, candy, and baked products, it is also found in pet foods. This is banned in Norway.

FD & C Green No. 3 (Fast Green) – This is one of the least used colors. You will find it in candies and beverages. In 1981, an industry sponsored study arose suspicions regarding bladder tumor, but FDA deemed it safe after re-evaluation. This has been banned in some European countries.

FD & C Yellow No. 6 (Sunset Yellow) – This had been shown to cause allergic reactions like hives, rhinitis (runny nose), and nasal congestion. It appeared to cause tumors of the kidney and adrenal glands in rats, and it may be carcinogenic. FDA reviewed studies on rats and believes that this color is safe to use. This color is banned in Norway and Sweden. It has been found used in sausages, candy, gelatin, and baked goods.

FD & C Yellow No. 5 (Tartrazine) – Aspirin-sensitive individuals usually react to tartrazine in the same way. This induces asthma, hives, and hyperactivity. Children consume more tartrazine containing foods than adults do, and unfortunately, this food color is suspected to cause behavioral problems among kids. According to the FDA, less than one out of 10,000 people may react to this additive in the form of hives. Therefore, the FDA has ruled that this color additive be declared on the label, so people sensitive to tartrazine or FD & C Yellow No. 5 can avoid it. This is found in candy, gelatin, beverages, baked goods, and pet foods.

FD & C Red No. 40 (Allura Red AC) – This is the newest red color additive to replace the other banned reds. It has undergone a lot of tests which were inconclusive and is still a suspected carcinogen. It is the most widely used food color and is mainly used in junk foods.

Cochineal (Carminic Acid or Carmine of Cochineal) – Cochineal is the bright red color that is obtained from tiny white bugs. These insects are raised by the millions in Peru and the Canary Islands. When crushed, its red color is extracted, and afterwards processed to destroy bacteria. It is used in fruit fillings, pasta, juice, yogurt, gums, other foods, and in lipstick. Cochineal is approved by the FDA, considered safe, and not required for listing on labels. It is non-certified or exempt from certification because it is a natural ingredient. It can cause allergic reactions.

Antibiotics, Hormones, and Pesticides

Food labels will not tell us about the presence of antibiotics, hormones, and pesticides in the foods we buy.

Antibiotics – About 40 percent of the manufactured antibiotics in the USA are used in feeds given to farm animals, such as fowls, cows, and pigs. Antibiotics and sulfa drugs are given routinely to these animals to prevent diseases.

Hormones – Hormones are mostly used in calves to stimulate growth and produce leaner meat. Diethylstilbestrol (DES) which caused cancer was banned for use in the USA in the late 1979. Nevertheless, some DES were still sold illegally until 1983. DES was later replaced with the sex hormones - estradiol, progesterone, and testosterone implanted in the ears of artificially raised cattle. While DES residues could be monitored, these new hormones cannot be detected. It is not different to the natural hormone already existing in the animal. The use of antibiotics and hormones came about as a result of commercial farming where farm animals are raised in factory-like pens. These animals are cooped up in areas so small that they could hardly move around – giving rise to infection and unsanitary conditions. In 1988, Sweden passed a law banning antibiotics and hormone and allowing cattle, pigs and chicken to roam freely within their confinement area. Sweden is a major producer of salmonella-free chickens in Europe.

Pesticides – Pesticide use started in the USA in 1800. The year 1943 marked the arrival of DDT, one of the major pesticides used in the USA against crop pests. DDT is not only cancer-causing but it is also neurotoxic. As a result of its damaging effect on wildlife and the environment, DDT was banned in 1972. The new pesticides manufactured later were not better than DDT. Later, these were also banned. Chemicals deemed to be safe were later proved to be harmful. It takes 20 years for the government to ban pesticides.

Pesticides, hormones, and antibiotics get into the body systems of the consumer in very small amounts, yet they can still cause considerable harm as they accumulate with time. In spite of the government ban on deadly pesticides, they still find their way into foods sold in the grocery stores. Manufacturers in the USA sell these pesticides to other countries that in turn use them on food they are processing and exporting into our country.

Fresh Produce Reportedly Containing the Most Pesticide

Strawberries	Bell peppers
Spinach	Cherries
Peaches	Celery
Apples	Apricot
Green beans	Grapes (imported)
Cucumber	Raisins
Potatoes	Peanuts

Fresh Produce Reportedly Containing the Least Pesticides

Alfalfa sprouts	Grapes (U.S.)
Asparagus	Avocado
Banana	Brussel sprouts
Cauliflower	Chives
Corn	Cranberry juice
Dates	Figs
Hazel nuts	Onion
Papaya	Pineapple
Shallots	Sunflower seeds
Sweet potato	Watercress
Watermelon seeds	Broccoli

Minimizing Consumption of Foods Containing Pesticides, Hormones, and Antibiotics

Buy fruits and vegetables in season and those produced in the USA.

➤ Keep a list of food manufacturers who abide by consumer-safe production and manufacturing techniques, and patronize them.

➤ Shift consumption pattern to organic produce sold from respectable supermarkets and reliable health stores.

➤ Buy lean meat or remove fat and skin from meat, as toxins reside mostly in fatty tissues.

Obviously, antibiotics, hormones, and pesticides will not be listed on labels. However, some producers who do not use any of these will make statements on their food packages, such as:

"This product is free from antibiotics, hormones, or pesticides"

See Appendix C, pages 224-225 for names of some producers providing:

➤ Meat products not using pesticides, antibiotics, and hormones
➤ Organic fruit juice
➤ Unbromated bread and flour products
➤ Organic rice

Food Allergy and Other Reactions

Food allergy is an adverse reaction of the immune system to food or food ingredients, that would otherwise be harmless to most. Additives are not the only substance that cause allergies. Whole foods can also provoke this. It is important to know if you or any member of your family is allergic to a certain substance. This can prevent any unpleasant or life-threatening event.

Symptoms of Food Allergy

➤ Swelling or itching of the mouth or throat
➤ Nausea
➤ Vomiting
➤ Diarrhea
➤ Stomach cramps
➤ Anaphylactic shock
➤ Itching
➤ Hives
➤ Skin rash or flushes
➤ Asthma

Some Foods That Cause Allergies

A number of foods cause allergies, but those commonly known to cause these are the following:

Some Foods That Cause Allergies	
Milk	Eggs
Shellfish	Fish
Peanuts	Soybeans
Wheat	Tomatoes
Chocolate	Corn
Yeast	

Some people who are allergic to aspirin can also be allergic to foods that contain salicylates, such as raisins and prunes.

Safety Measures in Food Allergy Cases

➤ For mild cases, keep a diary and write down what medications you take, and what you drink and eat, for four weeks. Write down allergy symptoms as they develop. You may then be able to determine what you are allergic to. You can then decide not to eat this food or foods for four weeks. If you are still not confident about being allergic to these certain foods, you can reintroduce these to your diet one at a time. When you do, start the diary process, once again.

➤ For non-emergency cases, consult a physician who is an allergist and immunologist.

➤ When allergy symptoms experienced in different parts of the body are happening all at once (such as hives, throat swelling, difficulty in breathing, and low blood pressure) – it is referred to as anaphylaxis or anaphylactic shock. Treat it like a medical emergency.

➤ For "How to Report Adverse Reactions and Other Problems With Products Regulated by FDA," see Appendix D, pages 226-233.

Other Reactions

Aside from allergies, there are other reactions that do not involve the immune system:

➤ Food poisoning – caused by bacterial contamination

➤ Food intolerance – caused by a lack of digestive enzymes

➤ Food toxicity – the nature of the food is such that it can cause harm or death to anyone

➤ Food sensitivities or unknown reactions – unexplained reactions that disappear when the person stops eating the food

Watch out for foods and ingredients that you or your children are allergic or sensitive to. For support groups or more information on this topic, see Appendix A (Private Associations), pages 220-221.

Banned Additives

At one time, these banned additives were considered safe. After complaints and later studies, they were then banned. Some banned additives:

➤ Agee (Nitrogen trichloride)
➤ Cinnamyl anthranilate
➤ Cobalt salts
➤ Coumarin
➤ Cyclamate
➤ Diethyl pyrocarbonate (DEPC)
➤ Dulcin (p-ethoxy-phenylurea)
➤ Ethylene glycol
➤ Monochloroacetic acid
➤ Nordihydroguaiaretic acid (NDGA)
➤ Oil of calamus
➤ Polyoxythylene-8-stearate (Myrj 45)
➤ Safrole
➤ Thiourea

Banned Artificial Colors	
Butter Yellow	Red 2
Green 1	Red 4
Green 2	Red 32
Orange 1	Sudan 1
Orange 2	Violet 1
Orange B	Yellow 1 & 2
Red 1	Yellow 3
Yellow 4	

Some Safe Additives

Alpha tocopherol (Vitamin E) – Derived from vegetable oils, it is an important nutrient and antioxidant. It is used to prevent oils from getting rancid.

Anise – A natural food used for flavoring foods and beverages.

Annato (Bixin, Norbixin) – Peach color derived from tropical tree seeds.

Apricot kernel oil – Used in salads, this is a source of cold-pressed oil.

Ascorbic acid, ascorbyl palmitate, and sodium ascorbate (Vitamin C) – A nutrient and effective antioxidant which prevents formation of nitrosamine. It is also a color and flavor stabilizer. Used in processed meats, apple juice, soft drinks, dry milk, and beer. Sodium ascorbate is a more soluble form.

Bioflavonoids – A natural ingredient that prevents harmful effects of oxidation, specially on Vitamin C. It is derived from citrus fruits and berries.

Carotene (alpha, beta, or gamma), and **Beta-apo-8'-carotene** – Converted to Vitamin A by the body, it is used as a nutrient and food coloring in butter, margarine, and shortening.

Calcium Pantothenate or **tricalcium phosphate** – provides the mineral, calcium.

Calcium stearoyl lactylate and **sodium stearoyl lactylate** – These are dough conditioners and strengtheners. They also act as whipping agents. Used in dough, whipped cream, and processed egg whites.

Casein and **sodium caseinate** – A thickening and stabilizing agent, casein and sodium caseinate contain the essential amino acids in protein. It is found in ice cream, sherbet, and coffee creamers.

Citric acid and **sodium citrate** – Citric acid is used as an antioxidant and as a fruity and tart flavoring. Sodium citrate is used as an emulsifier in ice cream. It is also used to control the acidity of fruit products such as gelatin, jams, and candies.

Grapeseed oil – Oil from grapeseeds is used for flavoring.

Cyanocobalamine – Provides Vitamin B-12.

Ergocalciferol – Provides Vitamin D.

Erythorbic acid – An antioxidant similar to ascorbic acid but with no vitamin value. Used also as a flavor and color stabilizer in meat products, baked foods, and beverages.

Ferrous gluconate – Used for color and flavor. Found in black olives and gives a uniform black hue. It is a good source of iron.

Fumaric acid – Derived from plant tissues and used as a tartness agent due to its high acidic quality. It remains solid at room temperature and used in pie fillings, powdered drinks, and gelatin desserts.

Gums – These are used in low fat foods, especially desserts as fat substitutes:

➤ **Furcelleran** – Derived from a seaweed, it is a stabilizer and emulsifier used to form gels for pudding.

➤ **Guar** – Derived from an Indian plant, it is used as a stabilizer and thickener in drinks.

➤ **Locust bean** – Otherwise known as carob bean or St John's bread, it is used as a flavoring in ice cream. It makes a good chocolate substitute.

➤ **Karaya** – Obtained from a tree in India and is used as flavoring in a lot of foods.

Lactic acid – It is produced by the fermentation of plant tissues and dairy whey. Lactic acid acts as an acid controller. It is also a flavor enhancer, a colorant, and a preservative. It is used in Spanish olives, cheese, carbonated drinks, and in frozen desserts.

Lactose – This is a carbohydrate in milk. It is used as a mild sweetener in pastries and whipped topping mix. Some Asians have lactose intolerance or trouble digesting it.

Lecithin – Contains a B-complex nutrient (choline) and acts as a fat emulsifier, preventing the separation of oil and water. It is also an antioxidant and used in margarine, ice cream, and baked foods.

Lemon balm – This is used as a flavoring for food.

Pectin – A stabilizer and thickener for dairy products and fruit preserves.

Potassium Ascorbate – Potassium salt of Vitamin C which acts as an antioxidant.

Potassium sorbate and **Sorbic acid** – Both are mold inhibitors and used in cheese, cheesecakes, salads, cake, wines, and dry fruits. Sorbic acid is also known as sorbistat, acetic acid, hedienic acid, and hexadienoic acid.

Salt (Sodium chloride) – Used in most food products as flavoring for processed foods, chips, soups, and crackers.

Sodium Riboflavin or **Riboflavin** – Used for its yellow color. This is known as Vitamin B-2.

Sugar (sucrose) – Used in most food products as a sweetener or as table sugar.

Turmeric – It is a medicinal root from India and Asia. It is used for its bright yellow color (curcumin) and is a flavoring in curries.

Zingerone – A compound that occurs naturally in ginger.

This additive listing is by no means exhaustive. Some people can still be allergic to a safe additive. Taken in excessive amounts, some safe additives can cause toxicity. Safe additives can become harmful if processing methods change its substance or quality, and if the process introduces a toxic by-product.

FOODBORNE ILLNESSES

Chapter

Foodborne Illness

Foodborne illness or food poisoning is a serious health problem resulting from eating contaminated food. In the United States, an enormous number of people fall ill from food contamination, resulting in severe symptoms, such as vomiting, diarrhea, asthma, paralysis, coma, or death. A variety of sources account for the origin of foodborne illnesses, most common of which are viruses, bacteria and other disease-causing organisms. Abiotic factors such as naturally occurring toxins, animal drug residues, pesticides, and environmental contaminants are also potentially able to cause illness. They either act singly or in combination, thus, aggravating the situation.

Foodborne Pathogenic Microorganisms and Natural Toxins

The Center for Food Safety and Applied Nutrition (CFSAN) prepared a handbook on foodborne pathogenic microorganisms (bacteria, viruses, and parasites) and natural toxins. This puts together the information on the subject from the Food & Drug Administration, the Centers for Disease Control & Prevention, the USDA Food Safety Inspection Service, and the National Institutes of Health.

List of Disease-Causing Organisms and Natural Toxins:

Pathogenic Bacteria

➤ *Salmonella* spp.
➤ *Clostridium botulinum*
➤ *Staphylococcus aureus*
➤ *Campylobacter jejuni*
➤ *Yersinia enterocolitica* and *Yersinia pseudotuberculosis*
➤ *Listeria monocytogenes*
➤ *Vibrio cholerae* O1
➤ *Vibrio cholerae* non-O1

➤ *Vibrio parahaemolyticus* and other vibrios
➤ *Vibrio vulnificus*
➤ *Clostridium perfringens*
➤ *Bacillus cereus*
➤ *Aeromonas hydrophila* and other spp.
➤ *Plesiomonas shigelloides*
➤ *Shigella* spp.
➤ Miscellaneous enterics
➤ *Streptococcus*
➤ Enterovirulent *Escherichia coli* Group (EEC Group)
   • *Echerichia coli* - enterotoxigenic (ETEC)
   • *Escherichia coli* - enteropathogenic (EPEC)
   • *Escherichia coli* O157:H7 - enterohemorrhagic (EHEC)
   • *Escherichia coli* - enteroinvasive (EIEC)

Parasitic Protozoa and Worms

➤ *Giardia lamblia*
➤ *Entamoeba histolytica*
➤ *Cryptosporidium parvum*
➤ *Cyclospora cayetanensis*
➤ *Anisakis* sp. and related worms
➤ *Diphyllobothrium* spp.
➤ *Nanophyetus* spp.
➤ *Eustrongylides* sp.
➤ *Acanthamoeba* and other free-living amoebae
➤ *Ascaris lumbricoides* and *Trichuris trichiura*

Viruses

➤ Hepatitis A virus
➤ Hepatitis E virus
➤ Rotavirus
➤ Norwalk virus group
➤ Other viral agents

Natural Toxins

➤ Ciguatera poisoning
➤ Shellfish toxins (PSP, DSP, NSP, ASP)
➤ Scombroid poisoning
➤ Tetrodotoxin (Pufferfish)
➤ Mushroom toxins
➤ Aflatoxins
➤ Pyrrolizidine alkaloids
➤ Phytohaemagglutinin (Red kidney bean poisoning)
➤ Grayanotoxin (Honey intoxication)

For more information, refer to Appendices E and F, pages 234-241:

➤ Onset, duration, and symptoms of foodborne illness
➤ A List of Food Product Recalls (from January to August 1999)

The Route of Food Contamination

Food contamination starts at the place where the food comes from and continues on to your dining table.

sea | cattle quarters | piggery | poultry | farm | orchard
▼
fishing vessels | slaughterhouse | packing houses
▼
trucks | freight trains
▼
warehouses | storage rooms | store shelves
▼
kitchen
▼
dining table

Aside from the above, a lot of of other factors can still add more contamination. The first four levels (from farm to store shelves) are under the control of the USDA, the FDA, the food producers, manufacturers, distributors, and the grocery store owners. The two government agencies, together with their federal and local counterparts, are responsible for monitoring food contamination. The private entities mentioned above play their part in making food available to consumers at a profit. The consumer's role in preventing food contamination is to:

➤ Take an influential role in food legislation;
➤ Report bad practices or non-implementation of regulations on food; and
➤ Observe safe handling, preparing, and cooking procedures. (See pages 211-213).

Food Products Likely to be Contaminated

➤ Foods that involve a lot of handling, thus passing through many hands
➤ Raw or uncooked red meats (beef, pork, mutton), chicken, and seafoods
➤ Foods in dented or partially opened containers
➤ Eggs, unpasteurized milk or juice, soft cheeses, and cream fillings
➤ Untreated water
➤ Salads, ready-to-heat foods
➤ Foods whose expiry date has elapsed
➤ Home-prepared foods

Special Populations Most Vulnerable to Foodborne Illness

➤ Children
➤ Elderly
➤ Pregnant women
➤ Immune impaired
➤ Allergic-prone
➤ Persons with liver, kidney, or stomach ailments, chronic disease, and those undergoing chemotherapy

How to Deal With Foodborne Illnesses
For Mild Cases

➤ Drink plenty of liquids - not tap water, but bottled water, Gatorade, or a sugary drink.
➤ Avoid solid foods and raw vegetables or fruits until you get over the illness.

When to See a Doctor

➤ Inability to hold down fluids
➤ Worsening abdominal cramps
➤ Bloody stools
➤ No improvement in symptoms after 24 hours
➤ High fever

When these symptoms are accompanied by vertigo, nausea, and difficulty in breathing or swallowing, progressive paralysis, or other serious symptoms - treat it as a medical emergency.

Reporting Problems with Food Products

If you want to report a problem with food products and want it to be investigated, prepare the following:

➤ **To Do**
   • Keep the original container or package
   • Keep the foreign object or cause of the problem (plastic, metal, insect, etc.)
   • Place the uneaten portion of the food in a plastic bag, put a warning sign, and freeze)

➤ **Contact Appropriate Agency**
   • For Meat, Poultry, and Egg Products: Call USDA Meat & Poultry Hotline 1-800-535-4555
   • For Restaurant Food: Call the Health Department in your city, county, or state
   • For Seafoods: Call FDA 1-800-332-4010
   • For Non-Meat Products: Check local phone book under U.S. Government Health & Human Services (for local FDA Office)

➤ **Prepare necessary information to give over the phone by writing it down. These are:**
  - Your name, address, and phone number
  - The brand name, product name, and manufacturer of the product
  - The size and package type
  - Can or package codes (not UPC barcodes) and dates
  - Establishment number (EST) usually found in the circle or shield near the "USDA passed and inspected " phrase
  - Name and location of store and date you purchased the product
  - If an injury or illness allegedly resulted from the use of a meat or poultry product, you will also need to tell the Hotline staff about the type, symptoms, time of occurrence and name of attending health professional (if applicable)
  - Make a list of everything you ate for he last ten days, including take-out and restaurant food

More Resources

➤ See Appendix A, pages 217-221 for addresses of government, medical, and private associations.
➤ See Appendix D, pages 226-233, How to Report Adverse Reactions and Other Problems With Products Regulatd by FDA
➤ Hotline for Foodborne Illness Victims: Call 1-800-350-STOP (Safe Tables Our Priority).

MACRONUTRIENTS

Chapter

Kinds of Nutrients

Food as a source of nutrient and fuel for the body, gives the impetus for human activities from the most basic to the most complex of functions. Nutrients are substances necessary for the nourishment and normal functioning of the body. Nutrients meet the body's energy needs for daily life, for growth and repair of body tissues, and for regulating vital physiological processes. The nutrients are *carbohydrates, proteins, fats, vitamins, minerals,* and *water.*

Carbohydrates, proteins, and fats are *macronutrients* that provide energy to the body. Vitamins and minerals do not provide energy. However, their presence, even in small but appropriate amounts, is vital for the release of energy to support the various body functions. Water, while considered as a nutrient in itself, renders the other nutrients in solution form. This makes the other nutrients available to different parts of the body.

Carbohydrates

The nutrient that is most readily available as a source of energy is carbohydrates. It provides fuel for the muscles (including the heart) and the nervous system. Carbohydrates also spare the use of protein which is used primarily for growth and tissue repair. The chemical structure of carbohydrates is based on a common unit – glucose or sugar. Carbohydrates are classified according to the number of sugar units. They differ only in the number of sugar units they have and how they are linked together:

➤ Monosaccharides – simple or single sugars
➤ Disaccharides – two monosaccharides
➤ Polysaccharides – complex molecules made up of multiple monosaccharides

Monosaccharides – These are simple carbohydrates made up of a single sugar molecule:

➤ Glucose – also known as dextrose, corn sugar, or grape sugar. Dietary glucose is less sweet than cane sugar or table sugar. Blood glucose or the glucose in our bloodstream is the form that carbohydrates take during digestion and absorption of starches in the body.

➤ Fructose – also known as levulose, or fruit sugar. It is sugar naturally occurring in fruits, vegetables, and honey. Fructose is much sweeter than table sugar and is not absorbed directly into the bloodstream.

➤ Galactose – this simple sugar is formed during the digestion of lactose or milk sugar.

Disaccharides – These are two monosaccharides linked together with the loss of a water molecule:

➤ Sucrose – this is our common table sugar, also known as cane sugar or beet sugar. It contains one unit of glucose and one unit of fructose. Vegetables and most fruits will contain, at least, some sucrose.

➤ Maltose – also known as malt sugar. It is formed during the breakdown of starch by digestion and in the germination of grains in the production of malt liquor, such as malt beer. It is found also in malted snacks and some breakfast cereals. It is made up of two glucose units.

➤ Lactose – also known as milk sugar. It is the only carbohydrate of animal origin. Lactose is made up of one unit of glucose and one unit of galactose. Persons who have low amounts of the enzyme lactase are called lactose-intolerant. They cannot digest lactose and might experience stomach cramps and diarrhea when ingesting milk or milk products, such as cheese, ice cream, yogurt, and cream (sour, whipped, half-and-half). It is less sweet than sucrose.

Polysaccharides or Complex Carbohydrates – These have several units of sugar strung together. It represents the starches and dietary fiber found mostly in fruits, vegetables, and grains:

➤Starches – Starch granules are covered by cell walls. When fresh, starches are difficult to digest. They have to be cooked so that the cell walls absorb water, expand, burst free, and become digestible. Starches are present in cereals, legumes, potatoes, corn, rice, pasta, bread, carrots, beets, squash, and other grains.

Starches can turn into sugars and sugars into starches. When fruits ripen, their starch turns into sugar. When sweet corn matures, it hardens, and its sugars turn into starches. Most simple sugars are absorbed readily in the bloodstream. Complex carbohydrates have to be converted to sugar (glucose) which takes longer for absorption in the body.

➤ Dietary Fiber – Dietary fibers are carbohydrates made up of the fibrous structure of palatable plants that remain undigested by the human stomach. Unlike cows and grazing animals, human beings lack the enzyme to digest fiber. Fiber in itself is not a nutrient and provides no vitamins or minerals. However, it is found in foods that contain a lot of nutrients such as grains, vegetables and fruits. Dietary fiber play a special role in promoting our health, and probably, in preventing some diseases.

Kinds of Dietary Fibers

Fibers are classified into *cellulose, hemicellulose, lignin, gums, pectin, mucilages,* and *bran.* They can also be grouped into *soluble* or *insoluble* fibers. A lot of foods contain both soluble and insoluble fibers, although some may contain more of one than the other. Dietary fiber is not available in foods of animal origin.

Insoluble Fibers – Insoluble fibers are the structural parts of plants. They do not dissolve in water, but hold on to water, giving bulk and softness to stools. This speeds up transit time of waste for excretion. Food waste that stays too long in the intestinal system produces toxins. These toxins re-enter the body inducing the formation of carcinogens. Insoluble fiber is known as "roughage" and act as "nature's broom."

Soluble Fibers – Soluble fibers are also found in plants. It dissolves in water and becomes viscous and mucilaginous. It binds with bile acids (cholesterol) and helps remove it from the body as waste.

Source of Dietary Fibers

Whole wheat	Peas	Oat bran
Almonds	Parsnip	Dried fig
Mustard greens	Cabbage	Oatmeal
Carrots	Okra	Popcorn
Strawberries	Eggplant	Rye bread
Barley	Green beans	Corn meal
White beans	Potatoes	Kidney beans
Black beans	Dried prune	Lima beans
Pinto beans	Dried date	Apple
Brussel sprouts	Raisin bran	Spinach
Citrus fruits	Bran flakes	Peanut
Cauliflower	Hummus dip	Pistachio
Broccoli	Whole grains	Dried apricot
Lentils	Pumpernickel bread	

Tips on Fiber Intake:

➤ If you are not used to eating adequate amounts of fiber and now want to start adding it to your diet, do this gradually in small amounts.

➤ Drink enough water to prevent constipation.

➤ Avoid excessive fiber intake and include other nutritious foods in your diet.

➤ To minimize intestinal gas or flatulence, see page 163.

Proteins

Proteins are composed of carbon, hydrogen, oxygen, and nitrogen. Some proteins also contain iron, phosphorus, and sulfur. Proteins are the second most abundant substance in the human body system (next to water) and constitutes about one-fifth of our body weight. They are made up of amino acids.

Amino Acids

Amino acids are the building blocks of protein. There may be hundreds of amino acids in a protein. These amino acids are linked together to form helixes, chains, spheres, and branched structures. Each protein has certain characteristics that are determined by the number, kind, and order of amino acids in its link. Amino acids can be classified into essential and non-essential amino acids.

Kinds of Amino Acids

Essential Amino Acids – These have to be supplied in the diet, as the body cannot manufacture them. These essential amino acids are as follows:

➤ Leucine – releases insulin and lowers blood sugar. It substitutes for glucose and acts as a healing agent for wounds.

➤ Isoleucine – plays a role in the conversion of energy, blood availability in the brain, and retains niacin.

➤ Valine – plays a role in the conversion of energy, repair of the brain myelin sheath, and influences neurological activities.

➤ Lysine – regulates calcium absorption and formation of collagen that forms bone, cartilage, and connective tissues.

➤ Threonine – an important constituent of collagen, controls fatty buildup in the liver when choline is inadequate, and plays a role in energy conversion.

➤ Tryptophan – regulates serotonin, a neurotransmitter that influences sleep and mood.

➤ Phenylalanine – manufactures norepinephrine, a neurotransmitter involved in learning, alertness, and memory. An antidepressant, it can alleviate pain and suppress appetite.

➤ Methionine – a source of sulfur for hairs and nails, increases lecithin production to limit fatty buildup, neutralizes toxins, and is an antidepressant.

➤ Histidine – chelates trace minerals and heavy metals from the body, reduces nervous tension, used in production of red and white blood cells, and plays a role in the cardiocirculatory process. It must be supplied in the diet to promote growth, and therefore, highly essential for children and infants.

Non-essential Amino Acids – These are equally important amino acids needed by the body. They are manufactured by the body and does not have to be supplied in the diet. The following are the recognized non-essential amino acids:

Non-Essential Amino Acids	
Arginine	Glutamine
Alanine	Glycine
Asparagine	Ornithin
Aspartic acid	Proline
Carnitine	Serine
Cysteine	Taurine
Cystine	Tyrosine
Glutamic acid	

The Role of DNA and RNA in Protein Synthesis

The DNA (deoxyribonucleic acid) controls the making of protein from amino acids. Each person is always different in some ways from another. DNA is the blueprint of an individual and contains the information about his cells, tissues, organs, or genetic makeup. The DNA gives the information to the RNA (ribonucleic acid) which then acts as a messenger or transport system. The RNA sees to it that the DNA is replicated in all the cells that compose the concerned tissue.

Kinds of Proteins

Complete Proteins – These are proteins that contain all the essential amino acids. These are found in proteins of animal origin (such as milk, eggs, and meat), except soybeans.

Incomplete Proteins – These are proteins that lack some of the essential amino acids. These are found in proteins of plant origin (like wheat, corn, rice, and legumes).

Some Functions of Proteins

➤ Growth, repair, and maintenance of cells and tissues in muscles, bones, hair, nails, and organs
➤ Production of enzymes, hormones, and chemicals that control body processes
➤ Regulate the maintenance of fluid and electrolyte balance – acidity, blood pressure, growth, blood sugar level, and metabolism
➤ Needed for transmission of impulses in the nervous system and making memory work
➤ Help in transporting nutrients and oxygen in the blood
➤ Formation of antibodies
➤ Enable blood to clot
➤ Serve as alternate energy source, in case carbohydrates and fats are not available

Sources of Protein

Meat, poultry, and dairy products are the best sources of complete protein. Strict vegetarians, who exclude even dairy products from their meals and are not knowledgeable on food combining, may become deficient in Vitamin B12 or Cobalamine. This can lead to anemia and nerve damage. However, without meat, one can still get complete proteins from vegetables and grains by learning to combine foods properly. For example – rice with beans, a slice of wheat bread with cheese, or potatoes with broccoli. Soybean is a vegetable whose protein content is comparable to animal protein. Soybean products such as "tofu" and "TSP" (textured soy protein), soy flour, or soy milk, are cholesterol-free meatless substitutes.

Sources of Protein

Animal Protein	Plant Protein
Lean meat	Dry beans
Poultry	Tofu
Fish	Nuts
Cheese	Seeds
Yogurt	Grains
Eggs	Lentil

Combining Foods to Get Complete Protein
(Combine a vegetable with a grain or pasta)

Vegetables	Grains/Pasta
Soybeans	Rice
White northern beans	Wheat
Lima beans	Corn
Kidney beans	Oats
Black-eyed peas	Barley
Chickpeas	Rye
Walnuts, almonds, peanuts *	Buckwheat
Lentils	Millet
Pinto beans	Noodles
Navy beans	Macaroni
	Spaghetti

*Use in small amounts because of high fat content.

Protein Requirements

The problem for Americans is how to limit excessive protein intake and how to determine protein of good quality. The body needs only a little protein to build and repair tissues. What it does not need will be stored as fat.

TABLE 1. *Recommended daily protein*

Age	Weight		Height		Protein
(yr)	(kg)	(lb)	(cm)	(in)	(g)
Infants					
0.0-0.5	6	13	60	24	13
0.5-1.0	9	20	71	28	14
Children					
1-3	13	29	90	35	16
4-6	20	44	112	44	24
7-10	28	62	132	52	28
Males					
11-14	45	99	157	62	45
15-18	66	145	176	69	59
19-24	72	160	177	70	58
25-50	79	174	176	70	63
54 +	77	170	173	68	63
Females					
11-14	46	101	157	62	46
15-18	55	120	163	64	44
19-24	58	128	164	65	46
25-50	63	138	163	64	50
50 +	65	143	160	63	50
Pregnant					60
Lactating:					
1-6 mo					65
2-6 mo					62

Source: http//www.nal.usda.gov/fnic/Dietary/rda.html, 8/15/98.

Fats

Like carbohydrates, fats are composed of carbon, hydrogen and oxygen. However, fats have more carbon and hydrogen, but less oxygen. Fats are concentrated forms of energy that provide twice as much calories than proteins or carbohydrates. In its liquid form, fats are known as oils. It is insoluble in water and soluble only in organic solvents such as ether and chloroform. However, it can be emulsified.

Dietary fats or fats in foods, when consumed and synthesized by the body, becomes a source of energy. It is converted into body tissue, or stored in the body as *adipose tissue* or *body fat*. Fats, whether in foods, in the body tissues or in the blood, consist mostly of triglycerides. Triglycerides are made up of three fatty acids and one molecule of glycerol (glycerine).

Functions of Fats

➤ Provide over half of the energy used in basal metabolism
➤ Protect and cushion the internal organs
➤ Provide warmth and insulation to the body
➤ Aid in calcium absorption
➤ Aid in absorption and digestion of oil soluble vitamins (A, D, E, and K)
➤ Work with other nutrients to perform life-supporting functions in every body cell
➤ Constituent of prostaglandins that help regulate cholesterol
➤ Help maintain balance of sex hormones
➤ Contribute to the texture and palatability of food, take longer to digest, and delay returns of hunger feelings
➤ It must be present in the conversion of carbohydrates and proteins to energy

Types of Dietary Fats

➤ Saturated fatty acids
➤ Unsaturated fatty acids
  • Monounsaturated fatty acids
  • Polyunsaturated fatty acids
    ✦ Omega 6
    ✦ Omega 3
➤ Trans fatty acids

Saturated Fatty Acids – Saturated fats remain solid at room temperature. Sources are fats from beef, pork, or poultry, either in the form of plain fat (tallow) or marbled meat. They come mainly from foods of animal origin. Exceptions are palm and coconut oil. A high intake of saturated fats is linked to an increase of cholesterol levels, which can lead to atherosclerosis and heart disease. These are not needed in the diet.

Unsaturated Fatty Acids – These remain liquid or soft at room temperature. Food sources are fats from plants, fish, or some seafoods. The types of unsaturated fatty acids are:

➤ *Monounsaturated fats* (oleic acid) – Monounsaturated fats are liquid at room temperature, but turn cloudy in the refrigerator. Some sources of monounsaturated fat are olive, canola, peanuts, sesame, and avocado oils. Most noteworthy is olive oil, which is believed to lower LDL while maintaining HDL cholesterol levels, or possibly increasing it.

➤ *Polyunsaturated fats* – Polyunsaturated fats are liquid at room temperature and in the refrigerator. Compared to other fats, they easily turn rancid. They appear to lower "bad" cholesterol levels. Food sources are soybean, canola, walnut, cottonseed, corn, flaxseed, safflower, sunflower, and sesame oils. Under polyunsaturated fats, there are two "essential fatty acids" worth knowing – **omega 6** and **omega 3.**

Trans fatty acids – Trans fatty acids are polyunsaturated fats that have been chemically changed through the process called hydrogenation (see page 40). Food sources are margarine, shortening, spreads, breads, crackers, cereals, fried foods, and some prepared or processed foods. Trans fatty acids occur in nature in rare instances and in negligible amounts.

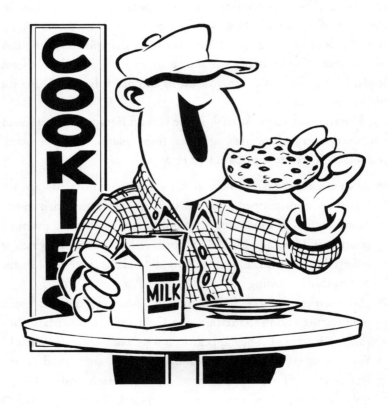

TABLE 2. *Percentage of fatty acids in fat sources* *

Fat/Oil	Monounsaturated	Polyunsaturated	Saturated
Olive oil	75	8	14
Canola oil	60	30	7
Soybean	23	58	14
Sesame	40	42	14
Walnut oil	23	63	9
Sunflower	20	66	10
Peanut oil	46	33	19
Hempseed	30	41	21
Corn oil	24	59	13
Safflower	12	75	9
Wheat germ	15	63	19
Flax seed	17	69	10
Coconut oil	6	2	89
Palm oil	39	9	50
Butter	24	3	51
Beef fat	32	36	71
Lard	45	11	39
Chicken fat	45	20	30
Margarine	21	18	8

*The fatty acids (monounsaturated, polyunsaturated and saturated) among the various fat sources in the above table, when added together, may not add up to 100%. Other substances present in the fats account for the difference.

All three types of dietary fats are present in most fats or oils. They vary in amounts and are mostly categorized according to the highest available amount of dietary fat present. Olive oils have more monounsaturated fats, and are categorized as such. Beef has more saturated fat, and therefore, classified as saturated fat.

Essential Fatty Acids

Two essential fatty acids that can make an impact on one's health are Omega 6 and Omega 3. These polyunsaturated oils are not only sources of energy, they are also constituents of body tissues, that should be added to the diet in appropriate amounts.

➤ The **Omega 6** Family:
  • Linoleic acid (LA)
  • Gamma linolenic acid (GLA)
  • Dihommo gamma linolenic acid (DHGLA)
  • Arachidonic acid (AA)
➤ The **Omega 3** Family:
  • Alpha linolenic acid (ALA)
  • Eicosapentaenoic acid (EPA) and Docosahexaenoic acid (DHA)

Prostaglandins

The other important function of Omega 6 and Omega 3 is its conversion into prostaglandins, which are essential to good health. Prostaglandins are hormone-like substances found in cell membranes exerting control on our metabolism.

Functions of Prostaglandins

Prostaglandin E1 (PGE1)

➤ Can reduce blood clots
➤ Relaxes blood vessels and bronchial tubes
➤ Lowers LDL cholesterol and triglycerides
➤ Boosts immune system
➤ Has anti-inflammatory action
➤ Thins the blood
➤ Stimulates vital hormone secretions
➤ Inhibits antacid secretion into the small intestines
➤ Suppresses insulin release from pancreas
➤ Alleviates depression
➤ Help kidneys in excreting sodium and fluids
➤ Regulates calcium and body metabolism
➤ Helps improve nerve transmission
➤ Inhibits PGE2

Prostaglandin E2 (PGE2)

➤ Increases blood platelet aggregation
➤ Causes inflammation
➤ Can increase tumor growth
➤ Constrict blood vessels
➤ Can cause water retention
➤ Increases pain

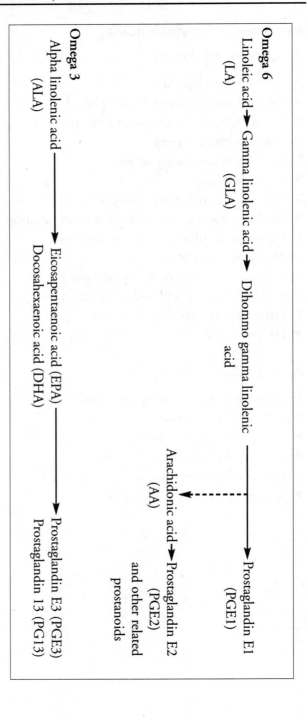

Figure 1

Conversion of Omega 6 and Omega 3 to Prostaglandins

Prostaglandin E3 and 13 (PGE3) and (PG13)

➤ Can reduce blood clots
➤ Has anti-inflammatory action
➤ Helps regulate blood pressure
➤ Boosts immune system
➤ Helps to lower and maintain triglycerides and blood cholesterol
➤ Enhances kidney function
➤ Regulates calcium and body metabolism
➤ Inhibits PGE2

Conversion of Linoleic acid (LA) to PGE1 and PGE2

The consumption of foods containing linoleic acid (LA) leads to its final conversion into prostaglandin E1 (PGE1). Before its final conversion, it first changes into gamma linolenic acid (GLA) and then into dihommo gamma linolenic acid (DHGLA).The pathway to PGE1 presents many obstacles which block its conversion. When this happens, it will instead convert to arachidonic acid (AA) which becomes Prostaglandin E2 (PGE2). The functions of PGE2, as one can see from the previous statements, are those we would like to avoid.

Conversion of Alpha linolenic acid (ALA) to PGE3 and PG13

When metabolized, foods containing alpha linolenic acid (ALA) converts to prostaglandin E3 (PGE3) and prostaglandin 13 (PG13). These prostaglandins are even better for the health than PGE1. Like linoleic acid (LA), the conversion of alpha linolenic acid (ALA) to PGE3 and PG13 has a lot of obstacles that could interfere with its conversion. When obstacles do happen, then the conversion to prostaglandins fails.

Factors that Block Prostaglandin Conversion

➤ Aging
➤ High blood cholesterol levels
➤ Elevated glucose or insulin
➤ Saturated fats
➤ Trans fatty acids
➤ Obesity
➤ Diabetes
➤ Smoking
➤ FD & C Yellow No. 5 (Tartrazine)
➤ Stress
➤ Caffeine
➤ Disease
➤ Alcohol

Factors that Facilitate Prostaglandin Conversion

➤ Vitamin C
➤ Vitamin B-3 and B-6
➤ Zinc
➤ Magnesium
➤ Essential amino acids (protein)
➤ Biotin

Food Sources of Some Essential Fatty Acids

Arachidonic acid (AA) is not only another by- product of conversion in the Omega 6 family metabolic pathway. It is also present in red meats, organ meats, egg yolks, and milk products. Because of the many factors that interfere with the conversion of LA and ALA to prostaglandins, health conscious individuals include in their diet foods already containing gamma linolenic acid (GLA) and eicosapentaenoic acid (EPA) as a short cut to prostaglandins.

Sources of Omega 6

➤ Linoleic Acid (LA) – corn, safflower, sunflower, walnut oils and wheat germ

➤ Gamma Linolenic Acid (GLA) – mother's milk, borage, evening primrose, and blackcurrant oils

➤ Dihommo Gamma Linolenic Acid (DHGLA) – not practically available

Sources of Omega 3

➤ Alpha Linolenic Acid (ALA) – flaxseed, smaller amounts in canola, hempseed, walnut, soybean oils, dark green leafy vegetables, and some beans

➤ Eicosapentaenoic Acid (EPA) and Docosahexaenoic Acid (DHA) – found mostly in cold deep seawater fish and some seafoods:

> ➤ Salmon – Atlantic, Chinook, Sockeye
> ➤ Tuna – Albacore, Bluefin
> ➤ Mackerel – Atlantic, King
> ➤ Norwegian sardine
> ➤ Pacific herring
> ➤ Cold-water halibut
> ➤ Anchovies
> ➤ Rainbow trout
> ➤ Striped bass
> ➤ Oysters
> ➤ Squid
> ➤ Swordfish
> ➤ Eel

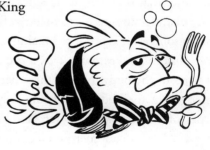

Some sources mentioned may contain both Omega 6 and Omega 3. It is listed as a *"source of"* when it contains more of that particular essential fatty acid. Some may contain only Omega 6 or only Omega 3.

Buying Dietary Fats

➤ To make sure that you buy edible fats or oils that still retain their essential fatty acids, buy products that are *"virgin,"* *"extra-virgin,"* *"expeller-pressed,"* or *"cold-pressed."*

➤ If they do not contain any kind of statement like those mentioned above, at least, look for a statement on food labels that the product was extracted *"without hexane"* or that it is *"free from hexane."* Hexane is a toxic and inflammable solvent.

➤ Choose to buy oils in bottles, specially dark ones, over those in tins or plastic.

➤ Avoid or minimize the purchase of lard or animal fat, hydrogenated vegetable oil, and coconut or palm oil.

➤ There ought to be more consumption of Omega 3 and less of Omega 6.

Cholesterol

Cholesterol is a type of sterol (steroid alcohol) – a waxy, fat-like substance that is present in all animal cells. It is essential to life. The body manufactures its own cholesterol from carbohydrates and other energy sources. It is produced mainly in the liver, and small amounts in the intestines. From the liver, it is circulated in the bloodstream to all parts of the body. Ninety three percent (93%) of the cholesterol is lodged in the body cells, while only 7% circulates in the blood. Types of cancer linked to fats and cholesterol are cancers of the prostate, breast, endometrium, colon, and rectum.

Dietary and Blood Cholesterol

Dietary Cholesterol – This is cholesterol found in foods of animal origin. It is not present in plant foods.

➤ Highest cholesterol content can be found in brains, egg yolks, kidneys, liver, and organ meats.

➤ Higher cholesterol content can be found in lamb, be
shrimp, crab, sardines, mackerel, and high fat dairy

➤ A slightly lower cholesterol content can be found
turkey, and lobster.

➤ The lowest cholesterol content can be found in most fish like
flounder, halibut, salmon, tuna, haddock, and some seafoods
(such as clams, scallops, and mussels).

Blood (Serum or Plasma) Cholesterol – This is cholesterol found
in our bloodstream.

Functions of Cholesterol

➤ Constituent of cell membranes
➤ Necessary for formation and function of nerve and brain cells
➤ Enables production of bile salts, Vitamin D, and adrenal steroid
hormones
➤ Aids in carbohydrate metabolism
➤ Essential to production of sex hormones
➤ Helps in fat digestion and absorption

Lipoproteins

Lipoproteins are a combination of fats and proteins. They act as
carriers or transportation for cholesterol in the blood.

Low-density lipoproteins (LDL) – The LDL's carry cholesterol
from the liver to the cells, through the bloodstream. Sometimes,
there is too much cholesterol that attach to the walls of blood vessels.
They pile up, forming plaques that make the walls narrower. A blood
clot blocking the narrowed blood vessel can lead to a heart attack or
a stroke, depending on the site where it occurs. LDL-cholesterol is
sometimes called the "bad cholesterol."

High-density lipoproteins (HDL) – The HDL's carry cholesterol away from the cells and bring it back to the liver. In the liver, it
is excreted as bile. High levels of HDL means a lower risk of heart
disease. HDL-cholesterol is sometimes called the "good cholesterol."

Blood Lipids

Triglycerides – Triglycerides are the storage form of fats that are found in the following:

➤ In foods, they are found as fatty acids such as: saturated, unsaturated, and trans fats
➤ In adipose tissue or commonly known as body fat
➤ In the blood or plasma

The cholesterol and triglycerides present in the blood-stream make up the blood lipids.

Cardiovascular Diseases (CVD)

Elevated cholesterol and triglyceride levels in the blood are some of the risk factors leading to cardiovascular diseases (CVD), namely:

➤ Arteriosclerosis – hardening of the arteries. *Atherosclerosis* is a form of arteriosclerosis involving the deposit of fatty plaques in the artery wall which thickens it and reduces blood supply to the organ
➤ Coronary artery disease (CAD) – hardening of the arteries of the heart reducing blood flow
➤ Heart attack (myocardial infarction) – obstruction of blood flow to the heart due to tissue damage
➤ Stroke – obstruction of blood flow to the brain due to tissue damage
➤ Peripheral vascular disease – circulatory disorder of the extremities
➤ Congestive heart failure (cardiomyopathy) – a disease of the heart muscle leading to malfunctioning of the heart

Risk Factors for Cardiovascular Disease

➤ Risk factors that one cannot change
  • over 55 years old
  • male sex
  • family history of heart disease
➤ Risk factors that one can change or modify
  • first-hand and second-hand tobacco smoking
  • high blood pressure or hypertension
  • physical inactivity
  • excess alcohol intake
  • obesity
  • diabetes mellitus
  • high blood cholesterol levels
  • high blood triglycerides
  • stress response

Information on how smoking contributes to cardiovascular disease and other ailments can be found in Appendix G, page 242.

Blood lipid Levels

Check Your Blood Lipid Levels

The blood lipid levels to check out are:

➤ Total blood cholesterol level
➤ High-density lipoprotein (HDL) level
➤ Low-density lipoprotein (LDL) level
➤ Triglycerides level

A high intake of saturated fats and dietary cholesterol can lead to elevated blood cholesterol and elevated blood triglyceride levels. As we know, elevated cholesterol and triglycerides are two of the risk factors for cardiovascular disease that we can change. To find out if you have these conditions, you have to take a cholesterol check in the clinic or hospital, where they will get your blood sample. The laboratory will then analyze your blood. It will be measured in terms of milligrams (mg) in one deciliter (dl) of blood. Other countries use the International System, with measurements in millimoles per liter (mmol/l).

Desirable Blood Lipid Levels

Blood Lipids	Desirable Levels
Total blood cholesterol	less that 200 mg/dl
LDL	less than 130 mg/dl
Blood triglycerides	less than 200 mg/dl
HDL	35 mg/dl or higher

For more details on blood lipid levels, see Appendix H, page 243.

The HDL-cholesterol measurement is just as important to know as the total blood cholesterol numbers. If your total blood cholesterol is higher than 200 mg/dl, but your HDL is higher than 35 mg/dl, your cholesterol level may not be that bad. It depends on the ratio of total cholesterol to your HDL. **A healthy ratio is 4.5 or 4.5:1. The ideal ratio is 3.5 or 3.5:1.** To get your ratio, divide your total cholesterol by your HDL.

Example:

Total Cholesterol is 250 mg/dl

HDL is 60 mg/dl

Ratio = 250 divided by 60

Ratio = 4.2 or 4.2:1

In the above example, although the total cholesterol seems to be unhealthy or above 200 mg/dl, the high HDL of 60 mg/dl manages to give this individual a healthy rating.

The triglyceride level tells us the amount of fat in the blood. Although triglyceride levels above 200 is considered high, yet physicians will prescribe medication only if it is over 800. Triglycerides, by itself, will not lead to heart disease, unless other risk factors are present.

The average adult can have a blood level test every 5 years. As of this writing, home cholesterol tests can only determine total cholesterol and not the other lipids. The home tests are useful if required by a physician for periodic testing in relation to a prescribed medication.

Blood Pressure, Cholesterol, and Sugar Levels

Fiber and the Fat/Cholesterol Diet

Diets high in fat and cholesterol are usually low in fiber. The introduction of high fiber foods in this kind of diet would minimize the harmful effects by:

➤ Absorbing fats and cancer-causing chemicals to dilute concentration
➤ Reducing stool transit time to minimize activity of harmful substances
➤ High fiber foods contain vitamins, minerals, and phytochemicals which inhibit or prevent cancer growth and improve the quality of blood

Fiber plays an important part in a fat/cholesterol diet when one is seeking to balance blood cholesterol and blood sugar levels.

Use Foods to Obtain Desirable Blood Pressure and Cholesterol Levels

➤ Eat foods that contain potassium, magnesium, calcium, and fiber
➤ Eat more of soybeans, fish or chicken (without the skin), and less of red meats, for protein
➤ Increase use of garlic, pepper, onions, herbs, and spices
➤ Decrease salt and sugar intake
➤ Choose whole grain breads and cereals, and other whole grain products, instead of refined flour products

➤ Avoid consumption and use of hydrogenated vegetable oils and saturated fats
➤ Ensure a daily diet of vegetables and fruits, that contain a variety of colors, specially dark green leafy vegetables
➤ Drink 6 to 8 glasses of water daily
➤ Avoid alcohol drinking and cigarette smoking
➤ Avoid drinking more than three cups of coffee per day

Aside from watching what you eat, there are other factors that can help one obtain a healthy blood pressure and cholesterol levels. Two important factors are **exercise** and **vitamin/herbal supplementation.**

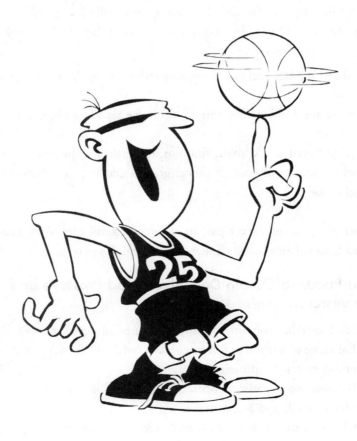

MICRONUTRIENTS

Chapter 5

Vitamins and Minerals

Vitamins and minerals are micronutrients because the body needs them only in small amounts. Nevertheless, macronutrients (carbohydrates, proteins, and fats) would not be able to perform their functions without them. Vitamins and minerals do not serve as fuel for energy, nor do they contain calories. However, they are essential for macronutrient utilization and have to be supplied in our diet. Vitamins are organic or chemical substances, while minerals are inorganic substances that are part of bones, teeth and nails. Both assist in enzymatic activities and act on the food we eat. *Vitamins and minerals in tablets or in artificial forms cannot take the place of food. They act as supplements.*

Vitamin and Mineral Deficiencies

Vitamins and minerals are taken through the foods we eat or as supplements in the form of capsules or tablets. To have a balanced diet, we need to eat a variety of nutritious foods. There are a few people who take the time and effort daily to buy, prepare, and cook this kind of ideal diet. The rest of the populace relies on canned, frozen and fast foods, or take-outs. Whatever way people get their food, they may still need supplements for the following reasons:

➤ Foods can lose some nutrients starting from production to processing, handling, storing, preparing, and cooking.

➤ Some bodies do not absorb or utilize nutrients as well as others.

➤ Environmental pollution in the form of cigarette smoke, air, and water pollutants – which we breathe and imbibe unknowingly – can cause nutrient losses and toxicity.

People Prone to Suffer Vitamin and Mineral Deficiency

➤ Dieters – These are people who stay too long on a restricted diet, people on diets which are below 800 calories, and those dieters who eat only one or two kinds of food for an extended length of time.

➤ Cigarette/cigar smokers and heavy drinkers.

➤ Drug users – These are users of addictive drugs, some prescription and non-prescription drugs, long term users of antibiotics, and birth control pill users.

➤ Some surgical patients, chronically ill people, and those suffering from a long-term or debilitating illness.

Some Signs of Vitamin and Mineral Deficiencies

Deficiency	Signs
Vitamin A	Night blindness, skin dryness, acne, and boils
Vitamin A, C, and Zinc	Decreased immune system
Vitamin B	Mental confusion, mood disorders
Vitamin B1	Muscle weakness/cramps, psychosis
Vitamin B2	Mouth sores or lesions, light sensitivity
Vitamin B3	Mouth sores or lesions, mental confusion or vertigo
Vitamin B6	Mouth sores or lesions, anemia
Vitamin B12, Folate, and Iron	Nerve damage, anemia
Vitamin C	Bruising easily, slow healing of wounds and fractures
Vitamin C and Folate	Bleeding gums
Vitamin C and Zinc	Skin healing problems
Vitamin D and Calcium	Softening of bones and teeth
Vitamin K	Uncontrolled bleeding
Fluoride	Dental decay
Iodine	Abnormal weight gain with puffiness in face, skin and hair dryness, overall weakness, and cold sensitivity
Magnesium and Potassium	Muscle weakness and tremors, Irregular heartbeats

Having the signs above should not necessarily exclude other causes or symptoms. The listing above purports to show evidence that vitamin and mineral deficiencies can affect one's health adversely.

Kinds of Vitamins

1. *Fat-Soluble Vitamins* – The fat-soluble vitamins are A, D, E, and K. They are not easily excreted and are stored in the liver and fatty tissues. Taken regularly in large amounts, they accumulate in the body and can become toxic.

2. *Water-Soluble Vitamins* – The water-soluble vitamins are C, B1, B2, B3, B5, B6, B12, Folic acid, and Biotin. The body takes the amount of vitamins that it needs and readily excretes the excess. Unlike the fat-soluble vitamins, there can be no toxicity, unless ingested in abnormally large amounts. These vitamins are easily destroyed by light and heat.

Fat-Soluble Vitamins

1. *Vitamin A* – preferable as beta-carotene (antioxidant)
   Sources:

   ➤ Yellow and orange colored fruits and vegetables, such as; oranges, cantaloupe, carrots, papaya, peaches, apricots, pumpkins, squash, sweet potatoes, mangoes
   ➤ Dark green colored vegetables, such as; broccoli, kale, collards, peas, watermelon, cherries, pepper, spinach, turnip greens
   ➤ Animal sources (retinol) like liver, egg, cheese, butter, milk

   Functions:

   ➤ Protects against xeropthalmia or night blindness (inability to see in the dark), strengthens and maintains health of eyesight
   ➤ Maintains good condition of mucous membranes, skin, and hair
   ➤ Aids immune system

➤ Promotes proper bone and teeth formation
➤ External application helps against boils and ulcers
➤ In the form of carotenoids, works as an antioxidant, minimizing risk for some cancers and aging diseases

2. *Vitamin D* – ergocalciferol, cholecalciferol, viosterol, ergosterol, or "sunshine vitamin"
   Sources:

➤ Sunlight, cod liver oil, egg yolk, liver, butter, salmon, herring, sardines, fish oils

Functions:

➤ Regulates absorption and mobilization of calcium and phosphorus which are necessary to normal bone growth and maintenance
➤ Works with Vitamins A and C to prevent colds

3. *Vitamin E* (tocopherol) – an antioxidant
   Sources:

➤ Wheat germ, nuts, vegetable oils, whole-grain cereals and bread, liver, green leafy vegetables, egg yolk, butter, asparagus, avocados

Functions:

➤ Works with Vitamin A to protect lungs against air pollution
➤ Protects body against free radical damage and toxic peroxides that can cause cancer and accelerate aging
➤ Prevents and dissolves blood clots while acting as a diuretic, thus, lowering blood pressure and easing leg cramps
➤ Aids in healing of wounds and burns

4. *Vitamin K* (Menadione, phylloquinone, menaquinone)
   Sources:

   ➤ Dark green vegetables (broccoli, kale, spinach, lettuce, cabbage, turnip greens) alfalfa, cauliflower, yogurt, kelp, milk, peas, potatoes, liver, cereals and grains

   Functions:

   ➤ Helps prevent hemorrhages and blood clotting
   ➤ Helps in maintaining healthy bones and healing of fractures

Water-Soluble Vitamins

1. *Vitamin C* (ascorbic acid, cevitamin acid) – an antioxidant.
   Sources:

   ➤ Citrus fruit, tomatoes, green peppers, potatoes, melon, guava, papaya, broccoli, strawberries, and other fresh fruits and vegetables

   Functions:

   ➤ Prevents scurvy (disease characterized by bleeding of gums, anemia, hemorrhaging, tender and swollen joints)
   ➤ Important in collagen formation in muscles, adipose tissue, bones, tendon, teeth, and skin
   ➤ Helps in the metabolism and utilization of amino acids and other nutrients
   ➤ Can prevent nitrosamine formation that cause cancer
   ➤ Boosts immune system, offering protection against bacterial and viral infection, including the common cold

2. *Vitamin B1*, (Thiamin, Thiamine)
   Sources:

   ➤ Pork, liver, oysters, beef, organ meats, whole or unrefined grains and cereals, brewers yeast, peas, nuts, beans, bran

   Functions:

   ➤ Prevents beriberi (disease characterized by leg pains, difficult breathing, fatigue, personality changes, rapid heartbeat, accumulation of fluids in the extremities, severe muscle wasting)
   ➤ Helps release energy from carbohydrates and converts carbohydrate to fats
   ➤ Aids in the normal functioning of the muscles, heart, and nervous system
   ➤ Helps prevent air or seasickness

3. *Vitamin B2* (Riboflavin)
   Sources:

   ➤ Liver, milk, kidney, meat, fish eggs, brewers yeast, dark green vegetables, whole grain bread, yogurt

   Functions:

   ➤ Assists in metabolizing carbohydrates, proteins, and fats
   ➤ Important in cellular growth – promotes healthy skin, hairs, and nails
   ➤ Helps maintain health of mucous membranes, thus, eliminating mouth and tongue sores
   ➤ Helps promote eye health
   ➤ Helps in the conversion of the amino acid tryptophan into niacin

4. *Niacin* (Vitamin B3) – Available as niacin or niacinamide. Nicotinic acid as a form of niacin, causes flushing. In the body, it converts to nicotinamide or niacinamide.

Sources:

> ➤ Organ meats, muscle meats, poultry, beans, milk, eggs, whole wheat products, brewers yeast, wheat germ, fish, nuts, avocado, date, prunes, figs, pasta

Functions:

> ➤ Prevents pellagra (symptoms are dermatitis, diarrhea and dementia)
> ➤ Works with thiamine and riboflavin in energy production
> ➤ Important in nervous system function
> ➤ Can help reduce mental confusion, dizziness or vertigo
> ➤ Increases circulation and lowers blood pressure
> ➤ Helps in promoting a healthy digestive system

5. *Vitamin B5* (Pantothenic Acid, Panthenol, Calcium Pantothenate)
Sources:

> ➤ Liver, kidney, heart, meat, chicken, eggs, fish, cheese, whole grain cereals and breads, avocado, cauliflower, peas, nuts, sweet potatoes, dates, other green vegetables

Functions:

> ➤ Helps in metabolizing carbohydrates, protein, and fats for energy
> ➤ Protects hemoglobin (protein in red blood cells)
> ➤ Assists in vital functions: normal growth, cellular and nervous system development, and formation of hormones
> ➤ Reduces adverse effects of antibiotics

6. *Vitamin B6* – a compound of Pyridoxine, Pyridoxal and Pyridoxamine

Sources:

➤ Meats, liver, kidney, poultry, fish, eggs, dried beans, peanuts, walnuts, avocado, cabbage, cauliflower, oats, blackstrap molasses, wheat germ, spinach, green beans, potatoes, bananas, green leafy vegetables

Functions:

➤ Promotes proper assimilation of fats and proteins
➤ Assists in formation of red blood cells
➤ Helps in conversion of tryptophan to niacin and serotonin, and glycogen to glucose
➤ Reduces morning sickness and some forms of neuritis in the extremities

7. *Vitamin B12* (Cobalamin, cyanocobalamin – red vitamin that contains cobalt, a mineral)

Sources:

➤ Liver, kidney, heart, oysters, clams, meat, eggs, milk, crab, salmon, sardines, yogurt, shrimp

Functions:

➤ Aids in the formation of red blood cells
➤ Assists in metabolizing fats, carbohydrates, and proteins
➤ Proper insulation of the myelin sheath for normal functioning of nerve transmissions
➤ Promotes growth and appetite in children
➤ Increases energy, concentration, and balance

8. *Folic Acid* – Folacin, Folate, Bc, Vitamin M, Pteroylglutamic acid
   Sources:

   ➤ Dark green leafy vegetables, carrots, kidney beans, asparagus, broccoli, cabbage, cauliflower, green peas, lima beans, avocado, apricot, wheat germ, brewers yeast, cantaloupe, sweet potatoes, liver, kidneys

   Functions:

   ➤ Necessary to the formation of red blood cells and genetic material
   ➤ Aids in protein metabolism
   ➤ Aids in preventing birth defects

9. *Biotin* – Coenzyme R, Vitamin H
   Sources:

   ➤ Liver, kidney, eggs yolks, milk, dark green vegetables, molasses, green beans, brown rice

   Functions:

   ➤ Assists in carbohydrate, fat, and protein metabolism
   ➤ Minimizes eczema and dermatitis
   ➤ Reduces zinc deficiency
   ➤ May help prevent graying of hair and baldness

Consumption of raw eggs can lead to loss of biotin.

Kinds of Minerals

Minerals in living things are inorganic substances that remain even though the living tissue is burnt. Heat and light cannot damage it, unlike vitamins. Minerals perform vital functions in the body and assist vitamins and other nutrients to perform their functions. It helps in the transport of oxygen to cells, form hemoglobin, regulate heartbeat, form bones and teeth, metabolize protein, and contract muscles.

Essential minerals are composed of macrominerals and microminerals (trace minerals). Macrominerals are needed in amounts larger than microminerals. Although microminerals are needed only in very small amounts, it is still as important to human functions as the macrominerals. Taking minerals in excess can be harmful. Minerals can work together, against each other, or compete with each other.

A. Macrominerals	B. Microminerals
Calcium	Chromium
Phosphorus	Copper
Magnesium	Fluoride
Sodium	Iodine
Chloride	Iron
Potassium	Manganese
Sulfur	Molybdemum
	Selenium
	Zinc

A. Macrominerals

1. *Calcium*
   Sources:

   ➤ Milk, cheese, yogurt, canned salmon and sardines, clams, oysters, dried beans, peas, soybeans, dark green leafy vegetables, kale, broccoli, collard greens, sunflower seeds, blackstrap molasses

   Functions:

   ➤ Provides structure, strength, and maintenance of bones and teeth
   ➤ Aids in transmission of nerve impulses
   ➤ Works with magnesium in activating muscle contraction, including heartbeat

➤ Plays an important role in blood clotting
➤ Integral part of extracellular fluids while regulating fluid balance

In the prevention of osteoporosis and heart health, calcium works best with magnesium, vitamin D, and boron. If taking calcium supplements in the form of pills, avoid those with dolomite or bone meal, to avoid contamination from lead and other toxic substances.

2. *Phosphorus*
   Sources:

   ➤ Meat, poultry, fish, eggs, nuts, seeds, milk, cheese, whole grains, legumes

   Functions:

   ➤ Plays important role in production and transfer of energy from carbohydrates, fats, and proteins
   ➤ Helps maintain acid-base balance in the body
   ➤ A component of bones and teeth
   ➤ Necessary to growth, maintenance, and repair of body tissues
   ➤ Part of genetic materials (DNA)

Phosphorus deficiency is not common. Most foods contain phosphorus, especially meat. Soft drinks are high in phosphorus. Unfortunately, too much of this mineral can lead to depletion of calcium.

3. *Magnesium*
   Sources:

   ➤ Dark green leafy vegetables, almonds, cashew, soybean, figs, bananas, whole grain cereals and breads, lemon, grapefruit, apples, okra, beans, oyster, fish, pumpkin seeds

Functions:

➤ Important to energy production, nerve, and muscle function
➤ Aids in removing excess ammonia from the body
➤ Prevents tooth decay
➤ Works as a mild tranquilizer in combination with calcium
➤ Helps promote normal functioning of cardiovascular, neuromuscular, and renal tissues

4. *Sodium*

Sources:

➤ Sodium (salt) occurs in most natural foods, and added to a lot of prepared and processed foods

Functions:

➤ Combines with chloride (to form sodium chloride) in regulating fluid volume and dissolved substances outside the cells
➤ Helps maintain acid-base balance in the body
➤ Assists in muscle contraction and nerve transmission functions
➤ Its capacity to retain water can help prevent dehydration or sunstroke

5. *Chloride* (chlorine)

Sources:

➤ Table salt, potassium chloride, kelp, olives, milk, meat, eggs, and foods of both animal and plant origin

Functions:

➤ Essential in regulating acid-base balance in digestion
➤ Assists liver in waste excretion
➤ Helps transmit nerve impulses
➤ Helps regulate fluids in body cells

6. *Potassium*

Sources:

➤ Bananas, orange juice, dried fruits, bran, peanut butter, potatoes, apricots, dried beans, cantaloupe, tomatoes, watercress, green leafy vegetables, mint leaves, sunflower seeds, lean meats, milk, legumes, citrus fruits

Functions:

➤ Works with sodium to maintain fluid balance and normal heart rhythms
➤ Important in nerve transmission and muscle contraction
➤ Important in protein and carbohydrate metabolism
➤ Helps maintain normal blood pressure

7. *Sulfur*

Sources:

➤ Meat, milk, poultry, eggs, fish, dried beans, wheat germ, peas, peanuts, clams, dried beans, cabbage

Functions:

➤ A necessary component of healthy hair, nails and skin
➤ Assists in regulating oxygen uptake for normal brain function
➤ Fights acne and other bacterial infections of the skin

B. Microminerals

1. *Chromium*

Sources:

➤ Meat, cheese, liver, pork kidney, chicken, clams, whole grain breads and cereals, brewers yeast, corn oil, dried beans, peanuts, shellfish, mushrooms, egg

Functions:

➤ Enhances insulin in sugar metabolism
➤ Aids in use of glucose for fatty acid production and energy

There is less chromium as one gets older.

2. *Copper*
  Sources:

➤ Whole grains, dried beans, peas, prunes, nuts, dark green leafy vegetables, cherries, legumes, fish, liver, kidney, shrimp, oyster, nuts, cocoa powder, sunflower seeds, mushrooms

Functions:

➤ Essential in formation of red blood cells
➤ Influences iron absorption and facilitates utilization of Vitamin C
➤ Aids in formation of bone and connective tissue
➤ Helps in producing energy in body cells
➤ Assists in maintaining the myelin sheath covering the nerve fibers
➤ Component of respiratory enzymes

3. *Fluorine* (Fluoride)
  Sources:

➤ Fluoridated drinking water

Functions:

➤ Necessary to formation and strength of bones and teeth
➤ Helps prevent tooth decay

Too much fluoride can lead to brown stains or discoloration of teeth.

4. *Iodine* (Iodide)

   Sources:

   ➤ Iodized salt, seafood, sea salt, saltwater fish, kelp, onions

   Functions:

   ➤ As a component of the thyroid hormone, it increases oxygen uptake, basal and energy metabolic rates
   ➤ Promotes mental alertness
   ➤ Influences growth and development

5. *Iron*

   Sources:

   ➤ Liver, organ meats, meat, dried fruits, lima beans, legumes, sardines, prune juice, oysters, dark green leafy vegetables, asparagus, molasses, oatmeal, eggs, shrimps, whole grain cereals, potatoes

   Functions:

   ➤ Component of hemoglobin in the blood and myoglobin in the muscles which carry and release oxygen
   ➤ Facilitates energy production needed for collagen synthesis
   ➤ Prevents anemia

Only a small percent of dietary iron is absorbed by the body. An even smaller percent is absorbed if the source is of plant origin. Absorption can be improved if iron-containing foods are eaten with foods that has Vitamin C. Inappropriate iron supplements are harmful to children.

5. *Manganese*
   Sources:

   ➤ Liver, kidney, meat, whole grain cereals, dark green leafy vegetables, peas, nuts, blueberries, legumes, tea, instant coffee, cocoa powder, strawberries, pineapple

   Functions:

   ➤ Helps activate enzymes that act on Biotin, B1, and Vitamin C
   ➤ Assists in metabolism of fatty acids, cholesterol, and proteins
   ➤ Assists in bone formation and development
   ➤ Important in manufacture of thyroxin

6. *Molybdenum*
   Sources:

   ➤ Dark green leafy vegetables, whole grains, legumes, liver, kidney and other organ meats, milk

   Functions:

   ➤ Essential to iron metabolism
   ➤ Helps prevent anemia
   ➤ Important in enzyme (xanthine oxidase and aldehyde oxidase) function

7. *Selenium*
   Sources:

   ➤ Wheat germ, bran, onions, tomato, broccoli, grains, garlic, milk, liver, kidney, meats, seafood, chicken

   Functions:

   ➤ Works synergistically with Vitamin E to delay aging and

hardening of tissues
➤ Binds to heavy metals, thus reducing toxicity
➤ Antioxidant properties may prevent cancer

8. *Zinc*
Sources:

➤ Pumpkin seeds, ground mustard, wheat germ, brewers yeast, herring, shellfish, milk, liver, meat, oysters, egg yolks, poultry

Functions:

➤ Plays an important role in enzymatic activities
➤ Important in:
  • treatment of acne
  • insulin activity and protein synthesis
  • immune system, taste, and healing of wounds
  • blood stability and maintenance of acid-alkaline balance
  • development and health maintenance of reproductive organs, specially the prostate

Recommended Dietary Allowances (RDA)

Recommended Dietary Allowances (RDA) are nutrient standards established for healthy individuals undergoing the usual environmental stresses. The committee on Dietary Allowances of the National Academy of Sciences (NAS) set up these standards as guidelines for the maintenance of good nutrition. The National Academy of Sciences was established by Congress more than a century ago, to provide professional and unbiased advice to the federal government. Members of this institute are experts in all areas of scientific and technological fields. See Appendix I, pages 244-245 for the RDA on vitamins and minerals.

Vitamin and Mineral Supplements

There is not one vitamin or mineral that is superior to others or one that can stand alone. They function as a team – some of them enhancing or assisting another, or limiting the function of the other vitamin, mineral, or enzyme. A marked deficiency in a vitamin or mineral can cause an ailment, or it can affect a person's emotional and mental stability. Deficiencies can cause depression, irritability, nervousness, lack of energy and mental alertness, among others. On the other hand, overdose or excessive intake of vitamins and mineral supplements in the form of pills can also lead to some unpleasant side effects like fatigue, weight gain, diarrhea, and hair loss. Megadoses of supplements can also cause serious harm in the form of kidney stones, liver, nerve damage, and even death. The basic way to get vitamins and minerals is through a healthy diet. If you think that you need supplements, consult a nutritionally-oriented (ortho-molecular) physician or registered dietitian. In addition, refer to books on vitamin supplementation.

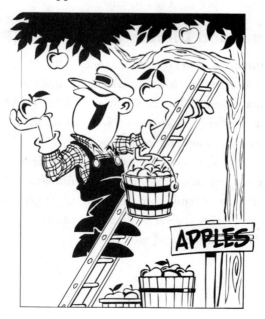

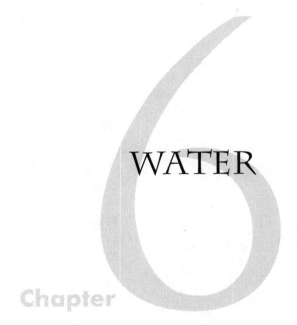

Chapter

WATER

How the Human Body Uses Water

As a substance necessary to life, water comes second to oxygen. Water is used by the body in several ways:

➤ Transport of nutrients and wastes
➤ Works as a medium or solvent for body secretions and excretions; such as – blood, urine, perspiration, and digestive juices
➤ Regulates body temperature
➤ Lubricates joint and body tissues

More Facts about Water

➤ It is more than 50% of the adult body weight and 70% that of an infant.
➤ A 10% loss of body water can be a health risk, while 20% can result in death.
➤ Daily requirement for drinking among adults is 6 to 8 glasses.
➤ Water has no calories.
➤ Water does not require digestion but it aids in the digestive process.

Contaminants in Water Supply

Lead

Most of it comes from corrosive lead plumbing. Copper plumbing is better, except when copper pipes contain lead soldering. Lead poison can lower a child's intelligence, cause high blood pressure, heart disease, and probably cause cancer, even at low levels.

Bacteria, protozoa, and viruses

Examples of these contaminants are *Escherichia coli*, *Giardia lamblia*, and *Cryptosporium*.

Industrial or Chemical Pollutants

➤ Pesticides, arsenic, and nitrates – These occur usually in rural agricultural areas using private wells. These chemicals are used in farms as pest eradicators and fertilizers.

➤ Asbestos – This causes cancer.

➤ VOC's (volatile organic chemicals) such as chloro-form, perchloroethylene, and trichloroethylene, vinyl chloride, tetrahydrofuran – these are neurotoxins and carcinogens. VOC's in the tap water can enter the body system through inhalation or absorption, when bathing or doing washing chores.

➤ THM's (trihalomethanes) – Chemicals formed by chlorine interaction with organic and carcinogenic pollutants. Some pollutants are decayed living things and other chemicals.

➤ Excess sodium – Some water may have hidden salts. This could be of importance to people who want to avoid it for health reasons.

➤ Radiation – in the form of uranium, radon, and radium. This may occur naturally in the environment or as a result of the contamination of water sources by nuclear plants releasing radioactive fission products.

Avoiding Water Pollutants

➤ First thing in the morning is to let the tap water run for at least 2 to 3 minutes (before using), to remove overnight lead accumulation.

➤ Put water in water filters, preferably in the evening.

➤ Use filters in showers and bathtubs.

➤ Install a water filter system.

➤ In the absence of drinking water filter, the alternative is bottled water.

Kinds of Bottled Water

➤ *"Spring-like," "spring fresh," "spring pure"* – These are plain filtered tap water.
➤ *"Mineral water"* – These are derived from natural springs with naturally occurring minerals.
➤ *"Spring water," "natural spring water"* – These are mineral water derived from springs with less mineral content and therefore has clearer taste.
➤ *"Distilled water," "purified water"* – This is water, boiled until it steams, leaving chemicals, minerals and impurities behind. It is then collected and condensed. It is tasteless, containing none of the desirable minerals the body needs. This is useful for medicinal, chemical, and pharmaceutical purposes.
➤ *"Sparkling water," "naturally carbonated," "naturally effervescent," "naturally sparkling"* – These are water that have naturally occurring gases coming from an underground spring.
➤ *"Club soda"* – This is tap water with added carbonation. It is usually high in sodium content than most bottled water.
➤ *"Seltzer"* – This is tap water filtered three times, with added carbonation, and nothing else.

Some Common Brands of Bottled Water

➤ Arrowhead Mountain Spring Water
➤ Calistoga Mineral Water
➤ Naya Spring Water
➤ Ozark Spring Water
➤ Sparkletts Crystal Fresh Drinking Water
➤ Vichy Springs Sparkling Mineral Water

Water Filtration Systems

There are a number of water filtration systems in the market. These systems have their own merits and demerits. Not one system is perfect for all intent and purposes. Filter units that attach to the faucet are but of minimal help. Water softeners introduced into the filtration system is suspected to remove calcium and magnesium – minerals essential to our health. A combination of reverse osmosis (RO) or ultra filtration and activated carbon filtration is acknowledged to serve most needs today.

Reverse osmosis filter removes a wide variety of contaminants like bacteria, PCB's, pesticides, uranium, radium, lead, and aluminum – but not chloroform and THM's. The use of cellulose membrane filters is preferred over polyamide in cases of highly chlorinated water. Installation of reverse osmosis filtration system is relatively expensive, while the filtration process is slow and wastes a lot of incoming water.

The use of *activated carbon filters* is considered as the oldest filtration system employed by most. It eliminates lead, radon, iodine, and phenols. It can also remove chloroform and THM's. It is generally recognized that granulated activated carbon filters are better than powdered ones. **In case of cartridge type filters, one should see to it that filters are changed on time.** Failure to do so can result in even higher levels of lead exposure, due to lead build-up in the filter.

Choice of Water Filtration System

The choice of water filtration system is conditioned by the quality of water to be filtered. To make a rational choice, it is important to have access to some basic data. Get the necessary information for decision making:

➤ Request for a water report from your local supplier regarding weekly and monthly measurements for VOC's, chloroform, aluminum, minerals, THM's, lead, other metals, alkalinity, radiation levels, bacteria, pesticides, total dissolved solids, nitrates, and industrial chemicals.

➤ Have your water tested by a private laboratory.

➤ Compare the results and, thereafter, decide what filtration system to use.

Refer to Appendix J, pages 246-261, for information on current Drinking Water Standards (contains list of specific contaminants and their enforceable and non-enforceable limits).

Conserve Water

➤ When shaving or brushing your teeth, do not let the water run continuously.
➤ In the shower:
  • Install low-pressure showerheads.
  • Take short showers.
  • Turn off the shower when applying soap or shampoo.
➤ Dishwashing:
  • When using the sink, fill it with water instead of letting the water run continuously.
  • Use the dishwasher only when full.
➤ Laundry:
  • Fill laundry basin or tub with water instead of letting the water run continuously.
  • Adjust water level according to wash load or use washing machine only when full.
➤ Outdoors:
  • Reduce water loss through evaporation by watering plants and lawn in the early morning or in the evening.
  • When washing the car, turn off the water hose, as needed.
  • Sweep driveways and sidewalks instead of using the water hose. Blowers are good alternatives.

Prevent Water Source Contamination

➤ Used oil, antifreeze, paints, and other toxic chemicals should not be poured into sewers or drains. They should be deposited in properly closed containers and turned over to the appropriate disposal system in the community.
➤ Use fertilizer and pesticides sparingly, and follow instructions.

➤ Pet litter, wastes, lawn, and garden debris should all be disposed off properly, and not into sewers or drains. These materials can cause fecal contamination.

➤ Provide ground covers, such as lawn grass or plants, to prevent instant water run-off (which may contain harmful chemicals) to sewers or drains.

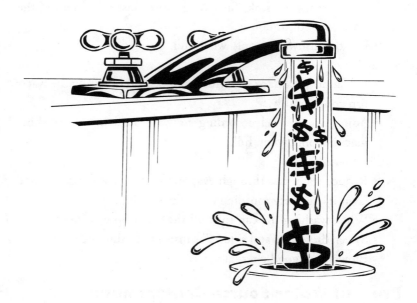

WEIGHT CONTROL

Chapter 7

Calories in Nutrients

Calories are the measurement of energy in the form of heat. It can refer to the amount of energy in food and to the amount of energy the body uses or "burns." Nutrients that provide energy are carbohydrates, fats, and proteins. They provide the following calories:

1 gram of carbohydrate = 4 calories
1 gram of protein = 4 calories
1 gram of fat = 9 calories

Fats yield roughly twice as much calories or energy than carbohydrates or proteins.

Calories and Alcoholic Drinks

Alcohol provides 7 calories per gram. Generally speaking, beer and wine contain insignificant amounts of nutrients, while the rest of the alcoholic drinks provide none. This is the reason why alcohol is said to provide "empty calories." Drinking in moderation is defined as one or two drinks a day. Four drinks a day is enough to cause damage to the organs in the body. Although moderate drinking is not harmful to most, it does not give any benefit either. The exception to this is red wine. Red wine, specially made from grapes, has been found to inhibit platelet aggregation in laboratory animals, thus preventing blood clot formations. This can be linked to a lowered risk for heart disease and possibly a reduction of LDL cholesterol. Good choices of red wine are those with labels that state, *"organic grapes,"* or *"without any added sulfites"*.

Who Should Not Take Alcoholic Drinks

➤ Children and teenagers
➤ Pregnant women or women trying to conceive
➤ People who plan to drive or report for work
➤ People taking prescription or over-the-counter medications

➤ People who cannot control their drinking
➤ Individuals whose work requires specialized skill and concentration, or attention to minute details

Effects of Immoderate Alcohol Drinking

Short-term effects:

➤ Reduced concentration and coordination
➤ Slow reflexes
➤ Slurred speech
➤ Blurred vision
➤ Sedation-depression of the central nervous system
➤ Increased perspiration and loss of body heat not felt by drinker
➤ Rob the drinker of these vitamins and minerals: thiamine, B2, niacin, B6, B12, folate, C, magnesium, potassium, and zinc
➤ May have life-threatening effect when taken with other drugs or medication
➤ Out of touch with reality and false psychological feelings of strength, warmth, bravado

Long range effects:

➤ Addiction to alcohol
➤ Personality change
➤ Shortened life expectancy
➤ Cirrhosis of the liver (hardening and inflammation of the liver leading to non-function, coma, and death)
➤ Sexual impotence
➤ Gradual deterioration of brain tissues leading to mental instability
➤ Damage to cells of the heart leading to heart failure
➤ Loss of interest in food may lead to peripheral neuritis (painful inflammation of the nerves) due to nutritional deficiency
➤ Increased risk for high blood pressure and stroke
➤ Increased risk for cancer
➤ Increased risk for osteoporosis (bones become brittle and fracture easily)

➤ Inflammation of the pancreas
➤ Interferes with fat metabolism

People have different physiological make-ups or body chemistry. Some can take more than two drinks without losing control of one's self. Others get undone with only one sip. Drinking on an empty stomach will only facilitate absorption of alcohol in the system. In spite of the high calorie content of alcohol, alcohol addiction is associated with malnutrition.

Basal Metabolic Rate (BMR)

Even at rest, the body uses energy from food for vital functions like digestion, cardiac and neural functions, body repair and maintenance. This energy expenditure at rest is the basal metabolic rate (BMR), expressed in calories.

Daily Caloric Allowance (DCA)

The calories we need to go through the day depend on our BMR plus the calories needed to perform the daily physical activities, like housework, driving, or exercise. These calories, added together, constitute our daily caloric allowance (DCA). To maintain our present weight, we just need to consume foods containing calories comparable or equal to our DCA.

TABLE 3. *Daily caloric allowance (DCA)*

Age	Range of Daily Calories Needed	
	Male	Female
4-6	1,300-2,300	1,300-2,300
7-10	1,600-3,300	1,600-3,300
11-14	2,300-3,700	1,500-3,000
15-18	2,100-3,900	1,200-3,000
19-27	2,500-3,300	1,700-2,500
23-50	2,300-3,100	1,600-2,400
51-75	2,000-2,800	1,400-2,000
75 +	1,650-2,450	1,200-2,000
Pregnant		+ 300
Lactating		+ 500

Daily caloric allowance (DCA) is based on several factors. Among them are gender, weight, age, activity level, internal and external body temperature, stress, amount of muscle and body fat. For these reasons, getting a precise DCA is difficult. Consult a registered dietician or physician if you are interested in getting a precise DCA. In the meantime, to give you an approximate idea of your own particular DCA, see Appendix K, pages 262-263.

Weight Control and Calories

Your own calculated DCA in Appendix K is based on your present weight and not your desirable weight. If you are one of the few who are at their desirable weight, then you just need to maintain your daily caloric intake and present activities. If you need to lose weight, then either or both of the following will help:

➤ Add or increase your activity level by exercise.
➤ Cut down on your caloric intake and/or reduce fatty foods from your diet.

A healthy weight loss should not be more than 2 pounds per week. More than that requires a doctor's supervision.

Decreasing Caloric Intake

When you decide to reduce your caloric intake, there are some important points to consider:

➤ Do not reduce calories by more than 300 per day.
➤ Total calories per day should not be lower than 1,200.
➤ Strive for a balanced diet of highly nutritious foods.

Being Overweight or Obese

A person is considered overweight if he is 20 to 40% above ideal weight and obese if 41% and above ideal weight. Exceptions to these are body builders who will weigh more, because muscles weigh more. Being overweight and obese places one in high risk for cardiovascular diseases and cancer. Those seriously pursuing weight loss cannot rely solely on the evidence of their body weight. They should also take into consideration the amount of their body fat. A person can be underweight and overfat, or overweight and not fat – at the same time.

Body Composition Tests

Body composition tests find out how much body fat you have. These tests usually determine not only your body fat, but also your lean meat and body water. Some popular body composition tests are as follows:

➤ Skinfold test – This test uses calipers to measure body fat by grasping and folding the skin in chosen sites.
➤ Hydrostatic weighing – This is only done in laboratories and requires being submerged in water while exhaling.
➤ Bioelectrical impedance analysis (BIA) – Electrodes are attached to extremities of the individual being tested and the analyzer machine estimates body composition.

➤ Near infra-red interactance (NIR) – Infra-red rays from a light
wand is placed on the bicep to determine body fat. This technology is similar to the grading of fat in meat sold in the supermarkets.

The body composition tests can be taken in fitness centers, clin-
ics, and hospitals. All body fat tests are not 100% accurate. It needs
the interpretation of a fitness expert; or the fulfillment of conditions
required by the test, from the individual being tested. If you do not
fancy body fat tests, the simplest way is to use a measuring tape or
put on a pair of old jeans. If you are eating the same kinds of food
and weigh the same, but your old jeans are tight, or your clothes-
measurements have increased – then you have gained fat.
Approximate suggested weight in terms of height and sex is provided in the next page.

TABLE 4. *Suggested weight for adults (in pounds)*
(without clothes and shoes)

Height	Male Average	Male Range	Female Average	Female Range
4'9"			102	95-117
4'10"			105	99-120
4'11"			107	101-123
5'0"	122	116-136	110	104-126
5'1"	124	118-138	113	107-129
5'2"	126	120-140	116	110-132
5'3"	129	123-142	119	113-135
5'4"	131	125-146	122	116-138
5'5"	134	128-149	125	119-142
5'6"	137	131-153	129	122-145
5'7"	140	134-157	133	126-149
5'8"	144	138-161	136	129-152
5'9"	148	141-164	140	133-156
5'10"	151	145-168	143	136-160
5'11"	155	148-172	147	140-164
6'0"	159	152-177	151	143-167
6'1"	163	156-181	155	146-170
6'2"	167	159-186		
6'3"	171	163-191		
6'4"	176	167-196		

Weight Loss, Fat Loss, and Health

When trying to lose weight, do not make weight loss as your only main objective. Your main goal should be to lose fat and attain the optimum health condition possible for you. An individual can be at his ideal weight and still be unhealthy, undernourished, or chronically sick. To achieve health is to have your bodily organs working properly so that you are of sound mind and body. You may still be healthy above your ideal weight (as long as it is not more than 10%);

or, if you are a body builder, have a large body frame or if you are big boned. Being overfat will put stress on your bodily organs and can lead to cancer, heart diseases, and other ailments.

To lose weight and maintain it, involves a healthy lifestyle. This means eating highly nutritious foods, avoiding high fat consumption, eating the right kinds of fats, regular exercise, a certain amount of self-discipline, and learning to deal with stress.

The "Wrong Ways" to Lose Weight:

➤ Lose weight only for a social event.
➤ Lose a lot of weight in a short time.
➤ Eat only one or two kinds of food.
➤ Starve yourself.
➤ No exercise.
➤ Rely only on weight-loss pills or weight-loss drinks.
➤ Deprive yourself of all foods that you like.
➤ Eat only once a day.

One or all of the above are temporary band-aids to what should be a permanent solution. After three months or less, the above activities will have to end because they are unrealistic and impractical. These can lead to health problems and more fat gain.

Carbohydrate-Protein Ratio Guide

Theories abound, creating controversies as to which ratio is healthier, or which one successfully induces weight loss. Some of the carbohydrate-protein ratios are:
➤ High carbohydrate-low protein ratio
➤ Moderate carbohydrate-moderate protein ratio
➤ High protein-low carbohydrate ratio
➤ "One nutrient only" diet (carbohydrate only or protein only)

High Carbohydrate-Low Protein Ratio

Based on FDA guidelines, an approximate percentage in terms of calories is shown below:

Legend:

(C) CARBOHYDRATES	**60%**
1. Fiber	5%
(P) PROTEINS	**10%**
(F) FATS	**30%**
2. Monounsaturated Fats	10%
3 Polyunsaturated Fats	10%
4. Saturated Fats	10%

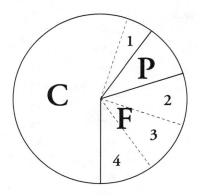

To calculate your daily carbohydrate, protein, and fat caloric allowances based on FDA guidelines, see Appendix M, pages 266-267.

The FDA guidelines should not be construed as a fixed regulation, but as a means to determine a comparative proportion.

Adjusting Fiber and Fat in the Diet

➤ One needs at least 5% of fiber for the daily caloric allowance. On the other hand, one should not take fiber in excess and forego other nutritious foods. Too much fiber can lead to a decrease in availability of some nutrients, because of its binding capability. However, the average American diet appears to suffer more from fiber deficiency rather than an excess.

➤ The 30% FDA recommendation for total fat in the daily diet should be seen as the maximum limit. It is better to go below this limit, especially in terms of saturated fat (striving for less than 10%). However, a zero-fat diet should not be attempted, unless medically prescribed. Fats are essential in synthesizing fat-soluble vitamins.

TABLE 5. *Daily fat allowances (in grams)**

Daily CalorieAllowance	Your Fat Allowance		
	30%*	20%*	10%*
1,200	40	27	13
1,300	43	29	14
1,400	47	31	16
1,500	50	33	17
1,600	53	36	18
1,700	57	38	19
1,800	60	40	20
1,900	63	42	21
2,000	67	44	22
2,100	70	47	23
2,200	73	49	24
2,300	75	51	26
2,400	80	53	27
2,500	83	56	28
2,600	87	58	29
2,700	90	60	30
2,800	94	62	31
2,900	97	64	32
3,000	100	67	33

Table 5 may not tally to the exact amount of the DRV in food labels due to rounding up of figures. Please remember that one gram of fat is equivalent to 9 calories.

The Weight Loss Problem

When trying to lose weight, one has to consider the short term, and specially the long term effects. An individual not losing weight on a high carbohydrate-low-protein diet, while doing regular exercise, needs to consider these factors:

➤ Some medications or supplements can cause weight gain.

➤ Individuals on the high carbohydrate-low protein diet may be doing the following things:

- Consuming carbohydrates in excess of their carbohydrate allowance.
- Consuming only carbohydrates of poor quality, like refined breads, sugared pastries, or carbohydrates that contain high fats and sugar.
- *Hyperinsulinemia* or *Insulin Resistance* can frustrate efforts to lose weight. Hyperinsulinemia is the presence of too much insulin in the blood because of:
  ✦ Too much production of insulin in the body
  ✦ The body resists taking in insulin into its cells, leaving insulin floating in the bloodstream
  ✦ A combination of insulin overproduction and insulin resistance

One of the causes of hyperinsulinemia is the excess consumption of refined or high glycemic carbohydrates which translates into glucose (sugar) in the body; or the consumption of just plain sugary foods. Done on a regular basis, it causes the body to crave more of it, leading to a vicious cycle. The symptoms are obesity, carbohydrate-sugar-fat addiction, high blood sugar, high blood pressure, and elevated total cholesterol.

Moderate Carbohydrate-Moderate Protein Ratio

If your diet consists of a high carbohydrate-low protein ratio which does not work in terms of weight loss, one can try the moderate protein-moderate carbohydrates ratio which can be modified, as follows:

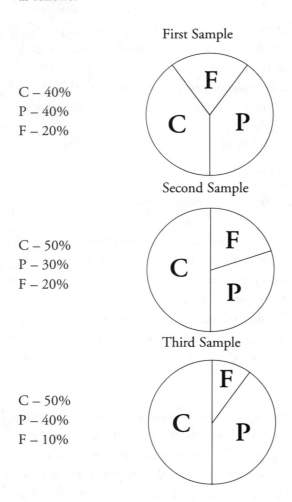

First Sample

C – 40%
P – 40%
F – 20%

Second Sample

C – 50%
P – 30%
F – 20%

Third Sample

C – 50%
P – 40%
F – 10%

Or you can try your own variation of carbohydrate, protein, and fat ratios.

Reminders on Diet Implementation

Our bodies and the way they work are all different. It is not practical to come up with a magic diet formula that will work for all. It may work for some, but there will always be some bodies that will react differently. When trying to find the right carbohydrate-protein proportion, try to bear these in mind:

➤ For protein sources – use poultry, fish, or beans. Eat less red meat.

➤ For carbohydrate sources – use whole grains, vegetables, fruits, and dietary fiber sources.

➤ For fat sources – use olive oil and omega 3 oils in appropriate amounts. Select low-fat foods.

➤ Avoid saturated fats and hydrogenated vegetable oils.

➤ Avoid artificial sweeteners, and minimize the use of sugars, sugary foods, and refined flour products.

➤ Include vegetables and fruits in your diet, everyday.

➤ Select a healthy diet you can live with on a permanent basis, and not just for a month or so.

It is important to pay attention to the healthful quality of the food, whether it is carbohydrate, protein or fats.

High Protein-Low Carbohydrate Ratio and "One Nutrient Only" Diet

The high protein-low carbohydrate ratio and "one nutrient only" diet cannot be a part of lifelong diets. Staying more than a month in these diets can be harmful to one's health. Health is compromised, especially if protein consumption relies solely on red meats. On these diets, one can only stay for 2 weeks or so. Afterwards, one has to go on to the moderate protein-moderate carbohydrate ratio. If this proportion is favorable, not only in terms of weight loss but also for health maintenance, then one can stay on this diet permanently. Otherwise, one needs to move on to the high carbohydrate-low protein diet.

HEALTH FOODS AND DIET CHOICES

Chapter 8

How to Take Charge of Your Diet

➤ Decide to take responsibility for a healthy diet because you make the ultimate decisions on what you and your family eat.

➤ Learn about matters relating to a healthy diet and keep abreast of new findings.

➤ Find out if your intake of essential nutrients is adequate.

➤ Be willing to change and adjust to a better and wiser food diet. Make small gradual changes.

➤ Plan a weekly or monthly menu based on a balanced diet and healthy food choices.

➤ Make a list of ingredients based on the planned menu as a guideline for grocery shopping.

➤ Read food labels and nutrient information on food packages.

➤ Keep a handy shopping guide in your pocket or handbag containing a list of harmful additives to avoid and a list of highly nutritious foods to buy, as your reference.

➤ Take an active role as a consumer in making your opinions and decisions known, on matters relating to better nutrition and food safety.

When you know more about the food you eat, you do not have to base your purchasing decisions only on advertisement, hype, and partisan agenda, which leave you open to exploitation and abuse, as a consumer. Instead, you will make informed decisions based on your own welfare and that of your family.

Keynotes of a Healthy Diet

➤ There is a lot of variety in food choices, in terms of color, texture, and nutrients

➤ Foods low in saturated fats and cholesterol

➤ Minimum consumption of sugar and refined carbohydrates

➤ Inclusion of complex carbohydrates, and whole-grains in the diet

➤ Contains right amount of dietary fiber

➤ Daily diet includes fruits and vegetables

➤ Emphasizes beans, fish, and chicken for protein source, while lean red meat is free from pesticides and hormones

➤ Foods that contain no harmful additives or preservatives

➤ Includes appropriate amount of monounsaturated oils and the right proportion of essential fatty acids (omega 3 and omega 6)

➤ Contains appropriate amounts of the essential nutrients

➤ Includes nutrient-dense and low glycemic foods

Looking For Quality in Foods

There are some characteristics or substances inherent in some foods that can create an impact on the body systems of an individual in terms of health maintenance and disease prevention. These are :

1. Nutrient Density
2. Low Glycemic Index
3. Antioxidants
4. Phytochemicals

1. Nutrient Density

Nutrient density is that quality of food wherein it contains a large amount of nutrients and very few calories. A calorie-dense food is the opposite, since the food contains more calories than nutrients. An example of a nutrient dense food is broccoli compared to a calorie-dense food such as doughnuts. Other nutrient dense foods are beans, green leafy vegetables, nightshades, peppers, onions, watercress, lettuce, and zucchini, among others.

2. Low Glycemic Index

Glycemic index is a relative measurement of how fast a carbohydrate is transformed into sugar and enters the bloodstream. A low glycemic index in a food would indicate that the food would tend to slow down or moderate the rise in blood sugar. Most low glycemic vegetables are beans, lentils, nuts and seeds, high fiber foods, and a few fruits. Whole foods, unaltered foods, and foods cooked for a shorter time usually have a low glycemic index. Foods with low glycemic index should be part of a diet that seeks to lower blood sugar levels.

Low Glycemic Foods:

black beans	cherries
black eyed pea	grapefruit
lima beans	pear
navy beans	plum
pinto beans	whole wheat noodle
kidney beans	peanuts
green peas	fruit sugars
chickpeas	apples
lentils	*cooked:*
soy beans	barley
milk	rice bran
yogurt	regular bran cereal

High glycemic foods are mostly sugary baked products like cakes, cookies, and doughnuts. Other high glycemic foods may include: vanilla wafers, rice cakes, instant cereals, most candies, white breads, instant or mashed potatoes, honey, raisins, and most instant foods.

3. Antioxidants

Antioxidants are nutrients or substances that provide body cells protection from oxidation caused by free radicals. Free radicals exist in the body, but get out of hand when more free radicals are formed by the normal burning of oxygen, by air pollution, X-rays, second-hand smoke, sun's ultra-violet rays, and other environmental pollutants. Antioxidants can protect the body by interfering with the oxidation of low-density lipoproteins (LDL), and may protect against some form of cancers and other degenerative diseases. Known antioxidants are beta-carotene (as a precursor to Vitamin A), Vitamin C, Vitamin E, selenium, and some phytochemicals from vegetables, fruits, and plant foods.

4. Phytochemicals

Phytochemicals are substances naturally occurring in plant foods that offer them protection from bacteria, viruses, and fungi. A single fruit or vegetable can contain hundreds of phytochemicals in trace amounts. Some of these also act as antioxidants. It was only recently that scientists took notice of phytochemicals and identified some of them. In the future, we will learn more about them and have a more standardized classification. By eating plant foods, we also avail of its phytochemicals which can protect us from cancer, heart disease, diabetes, eye problems, arthritis, osteoporosis, and other health problems of human beings.

Plants As Food

Plants as food contain not only the essential nutrients (carbohydrates, protein, fats, vitamins, minerals, and water), but also phytochemicals. If you or a family member is allergic or sensitive to some plant foods, it is worthwhile to know some plant food families.

Some Common Plant Food Families:

Apple: Apple, pear, quince

Alliaceae or Allium: garlic, onions, shallots, scallions, chives, leeks

Aster: artichoke, chicory, dandelion, endive, escarole, lettuce, sunflower seeds, tarragon

Blueberry: blueberry, cranberry, huckleberry, wintergreen

Brasicaeae (Cruciferae) or Mustard: broccoli, cabbage, cauliflower, brussel sprouts, chard, kale, collard greens, mustard greens

Buckwheat: buckwheat, garden sorrel, rhubarb

Cashew: cashew, mango, pistachio

Chocolate: cocoa, cola

Citrus: lemon, lime, orange, tangerine, citron, grapefruit, kumquat

Convulvulaceae or Morning Glory: sweet potato, water spinach or water convolvulus

Cucurbitaceae or Gourd: cucumber, muskmelon, cantaloupe, pumpkin, squash, bitter gourd

Fungus: mushroom, yeast

Ginger: ginger, turmeric, cardamom, galangal

Grains: wheat, barley, rye, rice, wild rice, oats, corn, millet, sorghum

Mint: mint, peppermint, spearmint, rosemary, sage, thyme, savory, balm, basil, horehound, catnip

Papilionaceae (Leguminosae) or Legume: peas, beans, soybean, winged bean, cowpea, and black eye bean

Solanaceae or Nightshade: potato, eggplant, tomato, pepper

Umbelliferae or Parsley: carrot, celery, and parsley

Walnut: English walnut, black walnut, hickory nut, pecan

General Classes of Phytochemicals

Carotenoids – Carotenoids are the most popular phytochemical of the Terpene family. Presently there are over 600 identified carotenoids, which contain red, orange, or yellow pigments. They are believed to protect against lung, colon, breast and prostate cancers; and promote eye and heart health. In the body, they convert to Vitamin A.

Flavanoids – There are more than 800 identified flavanoids at the present time. Flavanoids seem to act against bacteria and viruses, and block the action of carcinogens. These are anti-inflammatory and antihistaminic, reduce blood platelet aggregation, helpful in decreasing the risk of hypertension and heart attacks, and promote cellular health.

Organosulfurs – Organosulfurs inhibit cancer cell growth and nitrosamine formation, which triggers the beginning of cancer. Organolsulfurs are also antibacterial and antifungal.

A number of phytochemicals have been identified amongst several plant species. The following section is an attempt to enumerate some of these phytochemicals – their sources and their implied functions. This is not in any way complete. It will not be long before more information on phytochemicals come out in print, as new findings become available.

Phytochemicals, Sources and Their Functions

Anthocyanin/Anthocyanidin (flavanols)
  Sources:

  ➤ Grapes, currants, bilberries, blackberries, cherries, mangoes, figs, strawberries, eggplants, mung beans, soybeans, wheat, rice, kidney beans

  Functions:

  ➤ Antioxidant, inhibits tumor growth, prevents platelet aggregation and strengthens tissues and blood vessels, improves blood circulation and reduces blood cholesterol, promotes eye health, inactivates carcinogens

Beta-Carotene (carotenoid)
    Sources:

> Carrots, tomatoes, melons, pumpkins, squash, guavas, sweet potato, red cabbage, spinach, kale, mangoes, red peppers, cantaloupe, papaya, yellow squash, mandarin, orange, broccoli, spinach

Functions:

> Antioxidant, Vitamin A precursor, promotes heart health, reduces risk of cancer, stroke, and cataracts; resists effects of aging; promotes eye health

Capsicum (polyphenols)
    Sources:

> Hot Peppers:
  • Cascabel, cayenne, habanero, jalapeno, serrano
> Mild to moderate:
  • Anaheim, ancho, poblano, cherry, cascabel

Functions:

> Antioxidant, prevents formation of nitrosamines which lead to cancer, anti-inflammatory, minimizes pain, prevents blood clots and heart disease, increases metabolism, lowers cholesterol levels

Catechins (flavanols)
    Sources:

> Apples, grapes, green tea, avocado, bananas, cranberries, raspberries, strawberries, figs, peaches, plums, millet, black tea

Functions:

➤ Antioxidant, inhibits tumor production and carcinogenic activity, restricts rise of LDLs and triglycerides, anti-hypertensive

Curcumin (polyphenols)
Sources:

➤ Turmeric, curry powder

Functions:

➤ Antioxidant, promotes liver, stomach and gall-bladder health and good blood circulation, anti-bacterial and anti-inflammatory, lowers cholesterol levels, protects against cancer and heart disease, anti-fungal and anti-parasitic, more powerful than Vitamin E

Daidzein (isoflavones)
Sources:

➤ Soybeans, kudzu, soy products

Functions:

➤ Reduces risk of breast cancer by manipulating estrogen

Diallyl Sulfide (organosulfurs)
Sources:

➤ Allium vegetables: garlic, onions, scallions, chives

Functions:

➤ Inhibits nitrosamine formation and protects against initiation and multiplication of cancer cells; prevents platelet aggregation

Ellagic Acid (polyphenols)
Sources:

➤ Grapes, strawberries, raspberries, cranberries, apples, tea, walnut

Functions:

➤ Antioxidant, neutralize carcinogens (tobacco, air pollution, processed foods, barbecued meat) before they become potent; inhibits tumor growth

Genistein (isoflavones)
Sources:

➤ Soybeans, soy products, cruciferous vegetables

Functions:

➤ Weak estrogenic activity; anti-angiogenesis (prevents tumor and cancer cell growth), protects cell lining in blood vessels – preventing plaque build-up; helps decrease LDL, triglycerides, and total cholesterol

Glycyrrhizin (triterpene/carotenoid)
Sources:

➤ Licorice root

Functions:

➤ Inhibits estrogen-related tumors or cancers, anti-ulcer and anti-inflammatory functions; excessive intake can lead to a rise in blood pressure

Hesperidin (flavanoid)

Sources:

➤ Blossoms and peels of oranges, lemons and citrus fruits; tomatoes

Functions:

➤ Antioxidant, protects from capillary fragility, antiviral and anti-inflammatory, protects against allergies and cancer

Indoles

Sources:

➤ Cruciferous vegetables: broccoli, brussel sprouts, cauliflower, cabbage, kale, rutabaga, kohlrabi, turnips, mustard greens

Functions:

➤ Affects estrogen metabolism to protect against breast, colon, cervix, and lung cancers

Lentinan

Sources:

➤ Mushrooms: shiitake, oyster, portabello, enoki, black tree, fungus

Functions:

➤ Prevents platelet aggregation; boosts immune system; protects against bacterial, viral, and parasitic infections; inhibits tumor growth; lowers cholesterol levels

Lignans

Sources:

➤ Flaxseed, soybeans, sesame seeds, whole grains, legumes, walnuts, seaweeds

Functions:

➤ Antioxidant, promotes estrogen balance to protect against colon and breast cancer; anti-angiogenesis; inhibit cancers; may regulate cholesterol metabolism

Limonene (terpenes)

Sources:

➤ Rinds of oranges, lemons, limes, cardamom, garlic, coriander, mint, thyme, nutmeg, caraway, fennel seeds

Functions:

➤ Detoxify carcinogens in the liver and cause their excretion, inhibits cancerous growth in lungs and breast

Lutein (xanthophyll/carotenoid)

Sources:

➤ Dark green leafy vegetables (kale, spinach, mustard greens), dill, okra, peas, beet greens, broccoli, green beans

Functions:

➤ Antioxidant, protects against lung and reproductive cancers; protects against heart disease and macular degeneration

Lycopene (carotenoid)
  Sources:

  ➤ Tomatoes, red cabbage, guavas, pink grapefruit, dried apricots, tomato products, cranberries

  Functions:

  ➤ Antioxidant; linked to lower rates of stomach, lung, and prostrate cancers; protects against ultra-violet rays damage; reduces risk of heart disease

Phenolic Acids (flavanols)
  Source:

  ➤ Cruciferous vegetables, carrots, pepper, citrus, tomatoes, whole grains, berries, tea, squash, yams, parsley, herbs and spices

  Functions:

  ➤ Antioxidant, inhibits growth of cancer cells, inhibits platelet aggregation, anti-inflammatory

Proanthocyanidins (flavanols)
  Source:

  ➤ Grapes, raspberries, blackberries, figs, apples, avocados, bananas, plums, cornmeal, oats, millet

  Functions:

  ➤ (Same functions as anthocyanins)

Quercetin (flavanoid)
  Sources:

  ➤ Red grapes, red bell peppers, red raspberries, strawberries, cherries, cranberries, apples, bananas, broccoli, green beans, mung beans, barley, celery, green tea, tomatoes

Functions:

➤ Inhibits absorption and growth of cancer cells; anti-inflammatory and anti-allergy; prevents asthma, capillary fragility, cataracts, and macular degeneration

Rutin (flavanoid)
Sources:

➤ Buckwheat leaves, currants, asparagus, coriander, green tea

Functions:

➤ Antioxidant, antihistaminic, antiviral and anti-inflammatory; may protect against glaucoma, cataract, and diabetic retinopathy; prevents tumor, cancer, and capillary fragility

Soyasaponins (triterpene/carotenoid)
Sources:

➤ Soybeans, mung beans, kidney beans, peas, chickpeas, and other legumes

Functions:

➤ Antioxidant; inhibits estrogen-related cancers, like uterine, cervical and breast cancers; protects against fats and cholesterol-induced cancers; reduces circulating fats in the body

Sulforaphane (isothiocyanates)
Sources:

➤ Cruciferous vegetables

Functions:

➤ Helps liver to detoxify carcinogens and prevent tumor growth

Terpenes
> Sources:

➤ Oranges, grapefruit, lemons

Functions:

➤ Interferes with carcinogen activities; helps maintain healthy arteries; protects against damage to teeth and may prevent ulcer

Zeaxanthin (xanthophyll/carotenoid)
> Sources:

➤ Yellow corn, peaches, apricots, papaya, oranges, peas, prunes, dark green leafy vegetables

Functions:

➤ Antioxidant; acts like lutein to block blue light that damages the retina and help prevent macular degeneration; protects against cancer present in the blood and body fluids

Health Foods

Apples – High in soluble fibers and pectin, which help to stabilize blood sugar and lower blood cholesterol levels. May help to prevent atherosclerosis and heart disease. It has no saturated fat, sodium, or cholesterol and is low in calories. It helps maintain a healthy intestinal system and prevents constipation. It will help maintain healthy teeth and gums if eaten regularly.

Beans – Fiber and phytochemicals in beans lower "bad" cholesterol and triglyceride levels to prevent heart disease. Beans appear to lower the risk of colon cancer and other cancers, stabilize blood sugar, and helps prevent obesity. Aids waste elimination and maintains a healthy digestive system. Aside from fiber, it also contains proteins, iron, calcium, folate, vitamins A and B6, thiamine, potassium, and magnesium. Sources are adzuki, anasazi, pinto, navy, split peas, mung, lima, lentils, kidney, chickpeas (garbanzo), black-eyed peas and black turtle.

Berries – Some of these are blueberries, strawberries, bilberries (huckleberries), blackberries, cranberries, raspberries, boysenberries, loganberries, and ollalieberries. These are low in fat and sodium. They can help lower blood pressure. Their antioxidants and phytochemicals can help reduce the risk of cancer. As a good source of fiber, they can also reduce the incidence of colon cancer. Berries contain a lot of pectin, Vitamin C, and potassium. Cranberries have been used as home treatment for cystitis, and for prevention of kidney and bladder stones. Bilberries promote eye health.

Broccoli – May prevent tumors or inhibit their growth. Appears to reduce risk of cancers in the breast, cervix, prostate, bladder, colon, larynx, lungs, and esophagus. Contains bioflavanoids, fiber, calcium, folic acid, Vitamin C, iron, Vitamin A, natural laxatives, protein, and potassium.

Carrot – A source of beta-carotene, it is a precursor to Vitamin A. Decreases risk of skin, colon, bladder, and lung cancers. Boosts immune system. Helps lower cholesterol levels, prevents night blindness, and reduces risk of heart attack. Contains also dietary fiber and potassium.

Citrus – Appears to work against cancers, especially lung cancer, due to high Vitamin C and lemonoids content. May prevent cataracts and reduce the risk of heart disease. Contains soluble fiber, pectin, and glucarase that inhibit carcinogens and speed them out of the body. Sources are oranges, lemon, lime, kumquat, tangerine, and grapefruit. They are best eaten whole, rather than in juice form, to get all the advantages of its phytochemicals.

Cruciferous Vegetables – Help protect against estrogen-related and other forms of cancers. Its phytochemicals, beta-carotene, fiber, calcium, Vitamin C, iron, and folic acid contents, make this a nutrient-dense food. Sources are broccoli, arugula, bok choy, brussel sprouts, cauliflower, collards, kale, kohlrabi, mustard greens, watercress, radishes, turnips, rutabaga, broccoflower, and cabbage. Large intakes of raw cabbage is contraindicated for people with hypothyroidism. Otherwise, raw cabbage juice is believed to promote healing of peptic ulcers.

Fish – Omega-3 (fatty acids) in fish decreases the "bad" cholesterol levels and increases the levels of "good" cholesterol. It enhances the health of blood vessels and reduces the risk of heart attacks. It may relieve pain caused by rheumatoid arthritis. Rich sources are salmon, sardines, mackerel, tuna, and rainbow trout.

Garlic – Allium compounds in garlic seem to protect against cancer initiation and proliferation. It may lower cholesterol levels and blood pressure. It boosts the immune system, and prevents viral and bacterial infections. Nutrients found in garlic are selenium, vitamins A, B, C, and E, and allicin – an antibiotic.

Leafy Green Vegetables – Some leafy green vegetables or greens, are: kale, Swiss chard, collard, beet, chicory, mustard, turnip greens, and spinach. Greens help reduce cancer risk, control diabetes, lower cholesterol, and aid in weight loss. They are low in fats and calories. Aside from other phytochemicals, they also contain beta-carotene, vitamin C, fiber, chlorophyll, potassium, magnesium, and calcium. They are usually high in lutein and zeaxanthin that help protect against macular degeneration. It is an excellent source of folate.

Mushrooms – Mushrooms are fungus and are neither vegetable nor fruit. It contains canthaxanthin (a carotenoid) and lentinan, another powerful phytochemical. Mushrooms appear to have medicinal value, such as boosting the immune system, purifying the blood, strengthening the internal organs, lowering blood pressure and cholesterol levels; and protect against cancer. It also contains glutamic acid (a naturally occurring form of MSG), potassium, calcium, and selenium. Sources are portabello, reishi, shiitake, maitake, enoki, wood ear. Button mushrooms *(Agaricus)* are the least beneficial.

Non-Fat Yogurt – Yogurt is pasteurized milk with bacteria cultures. Lactose intolerant individuals can absorb yogurt better than regular milk. Low-fat yogurt is the better buy, but look at the list of ingredients, which says *"Lactobacillus acidophilus"* and *"bifidobacterium."* The word "active live cultures" is not sufficient. You have to check if one of the two bacteria *acidophilus* and *bifido* are specifically mentioned. A course of antibiotics can lead to yeast infection. A home treatment for this infection is taking plain yogurt daily, either as food, or topically. Yogurt as part of the diet may help protect against stomach and colon cancers. It is an excellent source of calcium, protein, riboflavin, and B12. It also contains vitamin A and folate. It may also help clear up one's complexion. Use it as a substitute for mayonnaise or sour cream.

Nuts and Seeds – Highly nutritious nuts and seeds are also high in calories and fats. Still, they contain a lot of phytochemicals, nutrients, and the essential fatty acids. In this category are chestnuts, almonds, pistachio, Brazil nuts, walnuts, macadamia, sunflower, pumpkin, sesame seeds, and cashew nuts. The best plant source of Omega-3 is flaxseed. These nuts and seeds help deactivate carcinogens, protect against heart disease, and help maintain healthy skin and hair. It may boost the immune system and lower cholesterol levels. Most of them also contain vitamin E, potassium, fibers, incomplete proteins, B vitamins, copper, selenium, calcium, magnesium, phosphorus, zinc, and iron.

Onions – It can prevent blood clots reducing the risk of heart attacks. Onions appear to raise HDL and prevent hypertension. Like garlic, it contains an antibiotic called allicin which is anti-inflammatory, analgesic, and anti-rheumatic. It also contains potassium. Green tops are good sources of vitamin C and beta-carotene.

Orange-Yellow Fruits – Orange-yellow fruits are cantaloupe, apricots, nectarine, pineapple, peaches, papaya, and mangoes. The beta-carotene and vitamin C antioxidants in these fruits help protect against cancer and other diseases. They are also a good source of potassium and pectin, which can help lower cholesterol levels.

Orange-Yellow Vegetables – The orange-yellow vegetables usually refer to some of the winter squash – acorn, buttercup, butternut, calabaza, pumpkin, and hubbard. Its rich color is an excellent source of beta-carotene. Aside from promoting heart health, its phytochemicals and antioxidants may protect against several cancers and help lower cholesterol. It appears to prevent and control lung cancer and also protects against second-hand smoke. It also contains Vitamin C, folate, potassium, soluble fiber, iron and calcium. Squash flowers and seeds are also edible. Noteworthy is pumpkin seeds, which contain zinc and protease inhibitors that seem to work against chronic prostatitis.

Peppers

➤ *Bell peppers* – This sweet variety of pepper is high in flavanoids and phenolic acids, which inhibit nitrosamine formation and prevent cancer. Its cancer-fighting sterols are precursors to Vitamin D. It is higher in Vitamin C than citrus fruits. The red peppers are even higher in Vitamins C and A than the green ones.

➤ *Chili peppers* – Related to the bell peppers, it contains capsaicin that can reduce pain and relieve nasal congestion. It may prevent blood clots to reduce the risk of heart attacks and stroke. It may also help increase metabolism and block cancer-causing compounds. Chilies are more nutritious than bell peppers. The red chili peppers are also higher in Vitamins C and A content than the green ones.

Red Grape Juice – Grape skins contain a naturally occurring fungicide called reservatrol that prevents clogging of arteries, helps lower blood cholesterol levels, but increases the good cholesterol. Reservatrol also shows some protection from cancer, it being an antioxidant, antimutagen, and induces cancer-blocking enzymatic activity. Other phytochemicals and antioxidant, especially quercetin and myricetin, are found in the skin, pulp, juice, seeds and stems from which grape juice is made of. These flavanols work in a way similar to reservatrol. They also contain pectin, iron, potassium, and Vitamin C. "Table grapes" or "organic grapes" will contain less reservatrol if sprayed with fungicides.

Spinach – Its phytochemical compounds help protect against lung and prostate cancer. Its beta-carotene, lutein and zeaxanthin protect us from macular degeneration. Its folate can help pregnant women protect the fetus from birth defects. It also contains Vitamin C, potassium, Vitamin B6, and riboflavin.

Sweet Potatoes – Neither a yam nor a potato, this root crop is rich in flavanoids, phenolic acids, and specially beta-carotene. It may help protect against uterine and lung cancers. It has almost the same benefits as carrots. It is also rich in Vitamin C, E, fiber, potassium, and iron.

Soybeans – Soybean contains complete proteins. It maintains estrogen balance and may inhibit ovarian and breast cancer. It helps build bone mass, reduces hot flushes, lowers LDL and total cholesterol levels, and reduces the risk of heart attack. It contains fiber, calcium, magnesium, potassium and iron. Soy protein in the form of tofu, tofuburgers, tempeh, textured soy protein (TSP) is a healthy meat substitute.

Tomatoes – Lycopene in tomatoes may protect against cancer, and specially prostate cancer. Tomato contains Vitamin C, beta carotene, B vitamins, potassium, and fiber.

Whole Grains – Fiber and complex carbohydrates are important constituents of whole grains. These can help prevent obesity and heart disease, at the same time, help control diabetes. It can also lower "bad" cholesterol and reduce the risk of colon and rectal cancers. As a source of incomplete proteins, they are low in fat and contain niacin, riboflavin, the B vitamins, selenium, folate, iron, and other vitamins and minerals. Sources are whole-wheat flour, oats, brown rice, barley, buckwheat (kosher), corn, millet, quinoa, whole-wheat pasta or noodles; whole wheat bread, muffins, and bagels.

Other Health Foods

➤ Bananas
➤ Beets
➤ Avocados
➤ Potatoes
➤ Plums
➤ Ginger
➤ Asparagus
➤ Celery
➤ Green beans
➤ Prunes
➤ Olive, sesame, and canola oils
➤ Artichokes
➤ Parsley, cilantro, watercress
➤ Okra
➤ Guavas
➤ Dried fruits
➤ Figs
➤ Skim milk
➤ Eggs
➤ Oysters and shellfish (if no allergies)
➤ Non-fat ricotta, cottage cheese, low-fat sapsago, part-skim mozarella

There are other health foods, aside from the ones listed. New findings in the future will bring them to our attention and we can add them to our list.

Abdominal Gas or Flatulence

Foods that usually cause flatulence are the following:
➤ Beans
➤ Cruciferous vegetables
➤ Carbonated beverages
➤ Dairy products
➤ Sweeteners – sorbitol, fructose, xylitol
➤ High-fiber foods
➤ Foods that one is allergic to
➤ Excessive intake of Vitamin C

Findings show that an average person passes gas more than 8 to 20 times a day, most of these possibly unnoticed. If not due to any medical disorder, bloating or smelly gas can be avoided or minimized by the following:

➤ *High fiber foods* – Increase fiber intake gradually to prevent diarrhea and bloating until your stomach adjusts.
➤ *Beans, cruciferous vegetables, and high fiber foods* – To these foods, add spices or other plants, such as: anise, peppermint, fennel, turmeric, ginger, bay leaf, horseradish, kelp or kombu seaweed, parsley, cilantro or coriander, cardamom, allspice, peppercorns, cayenne, and paprika.
➤ Use *"Beano"* which can be bought in supermarkets.
➤ *Dry beans* – Soak beans for at least 8 hours and discard water. Boil with new water until thoroughly cooked and tender.
➤ *Dairy products* – If lactose intolerant, use, *Lactaid* (available in supermarkets and pharmacies).
➤ Taking *"Lactobacillus acidophilus"* in yogurt or pill form helps minimize bloating and flatulence, maintains health and cleanliness of the intestinal system, if taken on a regular basis.

Meat

Meats are excellent sources of proteins. They also contain vitamin B12, riboflavin, thiamine, niacin, phosphorus, potassium, zinc, and iron. However, apart from nutrients, they also contain cholesterol and saturated fat. Meat choices are beef, veal, lamb, poultry, fish, and game meat. Under poultry, we have – chicken, turkey, Rock Cornish hen, duck, goose, guinea fowl, squab, pheasant, and quail. Poultry and fish have lower amounts of cholesterol and saturated fat.

Grading of Meat

The grading of meat has more to do with appearance than nutrient value. In beef, you can use it as a guide to fat content.

Major Grades of Beef

➤ *Prime* – tender, tastier, and juicy. It contains the most fat.
➤ *Choice* – More or less the same as Prime Beef, but with slightly less fat.
➤ *Select* – Not as juicy or flavorful as Prime and Choice, since it is leaner than the two.

Leaner Meat Cuts

➤ *Beef Cuts* – top round, tip round, eye of round, sirloin
➤ *Pork Cuts* – tenderloin
➤ *Lamb Cuts* – leg of lamb, sirloin chop, leg chop
➤ *Veal Cuts* – most cuts are leaner than beef, pork, and lamb
➤ *Poultry* – breast, drumstick. Aside from fat trimming, cooking without the skin can remove a considerable amount of fat. Dark meat has more fat and cholesterol than white meat.
➤ *Fish* – The fat in most fish can be a source of Omega 3.
➤ *Game meat* – Generally, they are leaner than other red meats.

Trimming fats off meat does not remove all fat since some of it are distributed throughout the lean tissue, specially in pork. It does help in lowering fat content.

USDA MAJOR FOOD GROUPS*

Guide to one adult food serving		
Food Group	One Serving	Servings Needed Daily
Bread, cereal, rice, and pasta	1 slice bread 1 oz ready-to-eat cereal 1/2 cup cooked cereal 1/2 cup cooked rice, or pasta 5-6 small crackers	6-11
Vegetables	1 cup raw leafy vegetables 1/2 cup chopped, raw, or cooked vegetables 3/4 cup vegetable juice	3-5
Fruits	1 medium piece of fresh fruit 1/2 cup of chopped fruit 3/4 cup of fruit juice	2-4
Milk Products	1 cup milk or yogurt 1.5 to 2 oz cheese	2-3
Meat,fish, poultry, dry beans, egg, and nut	2-3 oz of cooked lean meat, poultry or fish** 1/2 cup cooked dry beans 1 egg 2 tbsp peanut butter 1/3 cup nuts or seeds	2-3
Fats, Oils, sweets	Use sparingly	

*Adapted from "Food Guide Pyramids," U.S. Department of Agriculture.
**Eyeball method for assessing one serving size of these cooked meats is to compare it to a deck of cards.

Some foods like dry beans or nuts may fall either into the vegetable group, the meat group, or the oil group. If one counts it as a serving in one group, it cannot be counted in another group. Teen boys and active men can use the upper range in "servings needed daily." Less active women and older adults can use the lower range. Children, teen girls, active women, and less active men fall in the middle range of "servings needed daily."

FOOD GUIDE PYRAMIDS

Food pyramids are meant to be guides in making decisions about what types of meal or foods to eat. Five pyramids are shown to offer a broad choice for people of different ethnic backgrounds:

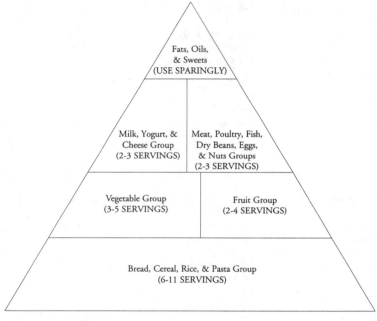

Figure 2
USDA food guide pyramid
Source: U.S. Department of Agriculture/U.S. Department of Health and Human Services.

The USDA Food Guide Pyramid is based on the recommended Major Food Groups for a daily diet. The other pyramids in the next pages have no recommended number of servings. Instead, they suggest some foods to be eaten daily, some weekly, and some monthly. Based on traditional ethnic cuisine, these food guide pyramids lead the way for more gustatory adventures in the food jungle.

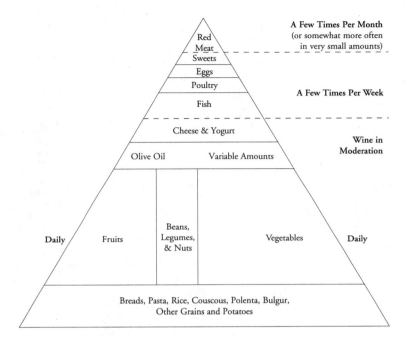

Figure 3

Mediterranean diet pyramid

Source: © 1994-1998 Oldways Preservation & Exchange Trust.

Mediterranean diet

➤ Carbohydrate sources are pasta, breads, and a variety of grains like – couscous, polenta, bulgur, and potatoes.

➤ This is high in monounsaturated fat, coming mainly from olive oil, which has been shown to promote health.

➤ The Mediterranean diet appears to increase the HDL (good cholesterol), and lower the LDL (bad cholesterol).

➤ Wine is drunk in moderation, with meals.

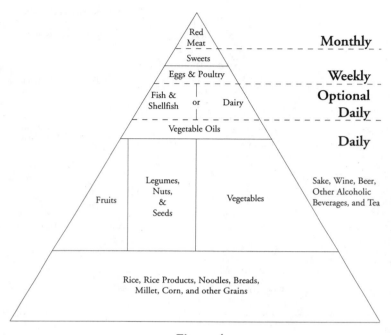

Figure 4
Asian diet pyramid
Source: © 1995-1998 Oldways Preservation & Exchange Trust.

Asian Diet

➤ Carbohydrate sources are rice and rice products, noodles, breads, millet, corn, and other grains.

➤ It is low in total fat content. Sesame oil is heat stable, and high in phytosterol that blocks cholesterol absorption.

➤ This diet appears to lower total cholesterol levels and may increase the HDL.

➤ Consumption of plant-based beverages, such as herbs, black and green tea, is part of the Asian diet.

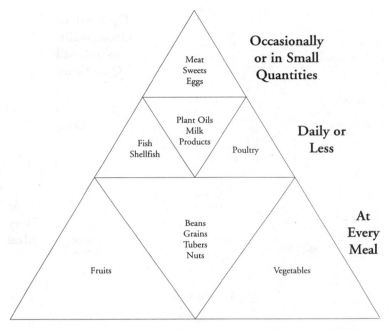

Figure 5
Latin American diet pyramid
Source: © 1996-1998 Oldways Preservation & Exchange Trust.

Latin American Diet

➤ Carbohydrate sources are beans, maize, potato, sweet potato, rice, taro, tortilla, breads, yucca, plantain, quinoa, peanuts, and legumes.

➤ Fat sources are obtained from consumption of nuts, vegetables, and fruits.

➤ There is a predominance of chilies in the daily diet.

➤ Hot chocolate drink is the daily beverage of choice.

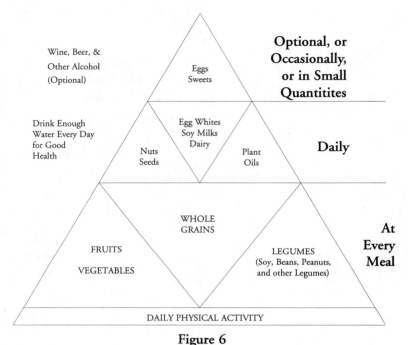

Figure 6
Vegetarian diet pyramid (Ovo-Lacto-Vegetarian)
Source: © 1997-1998 Oldways Preservation & Exchange Trust.

Vegetarian Diet

Vegetarian diets are generally considered meatless diets. However, there are many variations of vegetarianism. These are:

➤ *Vegan* – excludes all animal products
➤ *Fruitarian* – consists only of uncooked fruits, berries, and nuts
➤ *Macrobiotic* – includes fruits, vegetables, and high amounts of brown rice
➤ *Lacto-vegetarian* – includes fruits, vegetables and dairy products
➤ *Ovo-Lacto-Vegetarian* – includes fruits, vegetables, dairy products, and eggs

Aside from the above, there are other modifications of the vegetarian diet.

Advantages and Disadvantages of the Vegetarian Diet:

Advantages	Disadvantages
➤ Low in saturated fat	Could lead to deficiencies
➤ High in dietary fiber	in iron, Vitamin B12,
➤ High in antioxidants,	Vitamin D, and other
phytochemicals, and	nutrients
other nutrients	

When properly combined, vegetarian diets can provide complete proteins and balanced healthful meals. It can be delicious and tasty with the use of herbs and spices. A vegetarian needs to drink appropriate amounts of liquids due to the high fiber content of the diet.

Common Characteristics of Some Diets

The Mediterranean, Asian, and Latin American diets have these in common:

➤ Low in saturated fat
➤ High in complex carbohydrates and dietary fiber, as a result of the inclusion in the diet of fresh vegetables, fruits, and whole grains
➤ Plant foods are minimally processed
➤ Red meat is eaten sparingly in low amounts
➤ Low to moderate consumption of fish, eggs, poultry, and sweets
➤ Low to moderate consumption of milk and milk products

Asian countries, generally, have dairy-free diets. The exception are countries like India, Pakistan, Nepal, and Afghanistan who incorporate moderate amounts of yoghurt and homemade cheese products in their diet.

CHOOSE YOUR OWN FOOD GUIDE PYRAMID

The food guide pyramids previously mentioned are merely suggestions to facilitate food choices. Each pyramid can have variations. For example, Chinese, Japanese, and Indian cuisine are all lumped under Asian diet. Yet they can have a lot of differences in food sources, food preparation, cooking, and mixing of ingredients. There are still some ethnic diets that have not been included in our existing pyramids, like African, Middle-Eastern, and Polynesian diets. Decide on the pyramid of your choice, which you can adapt to your taste and preference. The preceding pages should have given you a lot of "food for thought" about healthy eating. Here are some suggested fun options:

➤ Use one type of pyramid this month and use another one the following month.

➤ Go lacto-vegetarian from Mondays to Fridays. On Saturdays, include fish in your diet. On Sundays include poultry or red meat.

➤ Make a combination of the different food guide pyramids and experiment on different tastes and physical appearances of foods.

PHYSICAL ACTIVITY

All the previously mentioned diets provide several nutrients to maintain and improve health. For optimal fitness, health experts strongly recommend combining good nutrition with physical activity in the form of regular exercise.

HOW TO READ FOOD LABELS

Chapter 9

Food Labeling Regulations

In accordance with the Nutrition Labeling and Education Act of 1990 (NLEA), the FDA set up regulations most of which went into effect in 1994. The regulations clarify doubts, previously arising in the past, from unfettered claims of food suppliers regarding their products. With these new regulations, it makes even more sense now to scan through the labels of food packages in the supermarket shelves. Food packages contain labels that offer useful and dependable information on nutrition to help the consumer make wiser food choices. Some important features of the FDA regulations on labels of packaged foods are the following:

➤ Serving sizes are standardized for similar products. These make nutritional comparisons easier.

➤ Almost all foods contain important nutrition information to impact one's health.

➤ The use of nutrient content descriptors such as "low-fat," "high fiber," or "sodium-free" can only be used if its nutrient level conforms to the uniform definition.

➤ Declaration of fruit juice percentages in juice drinks so the consumer will know if a grape-flavored drink actually has grape juice or not.

➤ A standardized format on nutrition information for customer convenience.

➤ Listing of all ingredients in foods containing two or more ingredients.

➤ Claims can be used on 10 scientifically proven relationships between a food (or nutrient) and the risk reduction of a disease.

➤ FDA certified color additives have to be mentioned by name.

➤ Sources of protein hydrolysates as flavors and flavor enhancers must be listed, since these contain MSG.

➤ Non-dairy foods which contain caseinate as a milk derivative must be listed.

➤ Implying a wrongful claim on the nutrient content of foods is prohibited.

Foods Not Included In The FDA Labeling Regulations

➤ Raw foods – meat (beef, pork, and poultry), fish, fresh vegetable, and fruits
➤ Foods served in restaurants, hospital cafeterias, airplanes, sidewalk vendors, vending machines, or foods that have to be eaten right away
➤ Foods that contain no significant amount of nutrients – plain coffee and tea, and some spices
➤ Individually packaged game meats, such as deer, rabbit, wild turkey, and ostrich
➤ Foods manufactured by small companies – employs less than 100 full-time employees and producing less than 100,000 units in a product line
➤ Ready-to-eat foods prepared in bakeries, deli, and candy stores
➤ Bulk foods that will have to be repackaged individually
➤ Medical foods prepared specifically for patients of special ailments
➤ Very small packages that do not allow space for nutritional information, although it must bear the company's name and address, or telephone number

Some companies producing the kinds of food listed above have started on their own accord to include nutritional information on their products.

Food Labels and Your Health

If you have health and weight problems, food labels can help:
➤ If you want to eat more fiber and calcium
➤ If you want to include Vitamins A and C in your diet
➤ If you want to avoid or eat less salt, sugar, cholesterol, and fats
➤ If you want to reduce the risk of some diseases

Major Parts of a Food Label

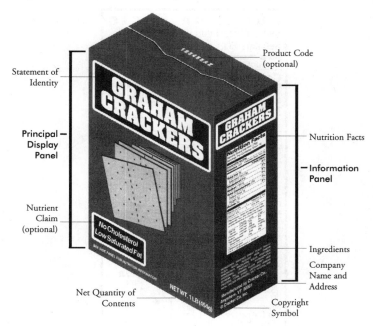

Figure 7

Major parts of a food package

➤ *Principal Display Panel* (PDP) – the front part of the package.
➤ *Information Panel* – Usually found to the right of the PDP. It contains the ingredients, calorie, and nutrition content values of the food in the package.

The Principal Display Panel

The Principal Display Panel (PDP) may contain the following:

➤ *Statement of identity* – identifies the name of the product
➤ *Nutrient claims* (optional)
➤ *Total contents in package* – quantity in pounds, grams, ounces, fluid ounces, or pints can be helpful in comparing prices. It does not include the package or wrapper it comes in.

Information Panel

Nutrition Facts		
Serving Size 1 cup (240mL)		
Servings Per Container about 2		
Amount Per Serving		
Calories 120		Calories from Fat 30
		% Daily Value*
Total Fat 3g		**5%**
Saturated Fat 1g		**5%**
Cholesterol 10mg		**3%**
Sodium 850mg		**35%**
Total Carbohydrate 18g		**6%**
Dietary Fiber 1g		**4%**
Sugars 1g		
Protein 4g		
Vitamin A 2%	•	Vitamin C 0%
Calcium 2%	•	Iron 4%

* Percent Daily Values are based on a 2,000 calorie diet.
Your daily values may be higher or lower depending on
your calorie needs:

	Calories:	2,000	2,500
Total Fat	Less than	65g	80g
Sat Fat	Less than	20g	25g
Cholesterol	Less than	300mg	300mg
Sodium	Less than	2,400mg	2,400mg
Total Carbohydrate		300g	375g
Dietary Fiber		25g	30g

Figure 8

Information panel

If the package is small or lack sufficient space, food packages may not follow the exact format of Figure 8.

Nutrition Facts

| **Nutrition Facts** |
| Serving Size 1 cup (240mL)
Servings Per Container about 2 |

Amount Per Serving	
Calories 120	Calories from Fat 30
	% Daily Value*
Total Fat 3g	**5%**
Saturated Fat 1g	**5%**
Cholesterol 10mg	**3%**
Sodium 850mg	**35%**
Total Carbohydrate 18g	**6%**
Dietary Fiber 1g	**4%**
Sugars 1g	
Protein 4g	

Figure 9

Nutrition Facts

Serving Size – the serving size, whether expressed in cups, table-spoon, or pieces – represent one serving.

Servings Per Container – This tells us how many servings are con-tained inside the food package, regardless of whether they come in packets or pieces.

Amount Per Serving – This represents:
➤ Total calories for one serving
➤ Total calories of fat for this one serving

Calories from fat are given importance because most of us need to lower our fat intake for health reasons. However, reduction of fat intake does not apply to children 4 years of age and below.

```
Nutrition Facts
Serving Size 1 cup (240mL)
Servings Per Container about 2

Amount Per Serving

Calories 120        Calories from Fat 30

                         % Daily Value*

Total Fat 3g                        5%
  Saturated Fat 1g                  5%
Cholesterol 10mg                    3%
Sodium 850mg                       35%
Total Carbohydrate 18g              6%
  Dietary Fiber 1g                  4%
  Sugars 1g
Protein 4g
```

Figure 10
Left hand column of "Nutrition Facts"
(one serving)

"Total fat" includes saturated, monounsaturated, polyunsaturated fats, and cholesterol if any. Saturated fat and cholesterol are especially mentioned in labels because of their contributory effect to cardiovascular disease.

Total "carbohydrates" would include sugars, complex carbohydrates, and dietary fibers. The amounts of dietary fibers and sugars are specifically stated because of their relation to health. Sugars include all types, including naturally occurring ones, such as fructose in fruits, and lactose in milk.

Percent Daily Values

The daily values are standardized for use on food labels. To come up with it, the FDA established two sets of reference values: the Reference Daily Intakes (RDI) and the Daily Reference Values (DRV).

➤ *Reference Daily Intakes* (RDI) – These are an average person's daily allowance of protein, vitamins, and minerals from food. It is based on the Recommended Dietary Allowances (RDA). The RDI can be seen in Appendix I, pages 264-265.

➤ *Daily Reference Values* (DRV) – Used as a consumer guide in food labels, these are daily allowances for nutrients and other food components related to health. The daily reference values for a 1,500, 2,000, and 2,500 caloric diet are shown below:

TABLE 6. *Daily Reference Values (DRV)*

Items Being Considered		Based on Caloric Diets of:		
		1500	2000	2500
Total Fat	less than	50g	65g	80g
Saturated fat	less than	15g	20g	25g
Cholesterol	less than	300g	300g	300g
Sodium (Salt)	less than	2400mg	2400mg	2400mg
Total Carbohydrate		225g	300g	375g
Dietary Fiber		20g	25g	30g
Potassium		3500mg	3500mg	3500mg
Protein		40g	50g	63g

➤ Allowance for fiber is 11.5 g for every 1,000 calories
➤ Cholesterol, sodium, and potassium stay the same for all caloric levels

Daily Cholesterol Intake

The total daily cholesterol allowance is less than 300 mg regardless of the daily caloric allowance. Since our body manufactures cholesterol, we do not really need a lot in our diet.

Here are 3 approximate scenarios of how one can easily go beyond the 300 mg limit for cholesterol:

Scenario # 1:

1 egg yolk	= 250 mg cholesterol
1 cup milk	= 35 mg cholesterol
1 tbsp butter	= 35 mg cholesterol
Total	= 320 mg cholesterol

Scenario #2:

6 oz chicken	= 132 mg cholesterol
6 oz tuna	= 108 mg cholesterol
2 oz cheese	= 60 mg cholesterol
Total	= 300 mg cholesterol

Scenario # 3:.

6 oz beef	= 180 mg cholesterol
6 oz shrimp	= 240 mg cholesterol
Total	= 420 mg cholesterol

Not putting a thought to what one ingests, can easily lead to an excess of cholesterol intake beyond ones daily allowance, even in just one meal. Apparently, the American diet does not suffer from cholesterol deficiency.

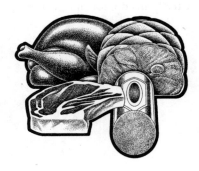

Percent (%) Daily Value

Nutrition Facts
Serving Size 2 oz (56g) About 1/4 cup
Servings Per Container 6

Amount Per Serving

Calories 120   Calories from Fat 60

	% Daily Value*
Total Fat 7g	**11%**
Saturated Fat 3g	**14%**
Cholesterol 50mg	**16%**
Sodium 490mg	**20%**
Total Carbohydrate 0g	**0%**
Protein 15g	
Iron	8%

DAILY REFERENCE VALUES:
* Percent Daily Values are based on a 2,000 Calorie Diet

	Calories:	2,000
Total Fat	Less than	65g
Sat Fat	Less than	20g
Cholesterol	Less than	300mg
Sodium	Less than	2,400mg
Total Carbohydrate		300g
Dietary Fiber		25g

Figure 11
"% daily value" (Sample No.1)
(canned beef)

The "% Daily Value" appears on the right hand column of the food label above and represents the percentage of a food nutrient on a 2,000 daily calorie diet only.

The daily reference value of total fat (see lower portion of the food label sample) for a person on a 2,000 daily calorie diet is less than 65 g. One serving of the canned beef shows 7 g of total fat which is equal to 11% daily value of 65 g. This person will have a balance of 58 g or 89% daily value of total fat. This balance can be met by servings from other food products, unless one consumes more than one serving of this food.

How about a person who is not on a 2,000 calorie diet? He can still use the "% daily value" for comparison on nutrient content, between one food product and another.

Compare the % daily value of "Total Fat" in Label Sample No. 1 (Fig. 11) and Label Sample No.2 (Fig. 12):

➤ If you are on a low fat diet, the label below is the better choice regardless of whether you are on a 2,000 calorie diet or not.

Nutrition Facts	
Serving Size 1/2 cup (140g)	
Servings Per Container 12	
Amount Per Serving	
Calories 170	Calories from Fat 25
	% Daily Value*
Total Fat 3g	**5%**
Saturated Fat 0g	**0%**
Cholesterol 0mg	**0%**
Sodium 15mg	**1%**
Total Carbohydrate 30g	**10%**
Dietary Fiber 6g	**24%**
Sugars 0g	
Protein 6g	
Vitamin A 0% • Vitamin C 0%	
Calcium 2% • Iron 8%	

Figure 12
"% daily food value" (Sample No. 2)
(mixed grains)

➤ If you are on a low sodium diet, you can see that Sample No.2 has less sodium.

➤ Notice, also, that the serving size of Sample No. 1 is only 1/4 cup, while Sample No.2 has a serving size of 1/2 cup.

You can then go on to make comparisons between food products, for other components; like fiber, sugar, or cholesterol, depending on your diet objectives.

Ingredients

INGREDIENTS: TOMATO CONCENTRATE MADE FROM RIPE TOMATOES, DISTILLED VINEGAR, HIGH FRUCTOSE CORN SYRUP, CORN SYRUP, SALT, ONION POWDER, SPICE, NATURAL FLAVORING

Sample of "Ingredients"

The first ingredient listed has the most amount and the last ingredient has the least. In the above example, tomato concentrate would be the main ingredient or the substance with the most quantity found in the food. Natural flavoring would be the smallest amount in this food item.

If sugar is the first ingredient, this means that the food would probably be of poor quality, containing a lot of calories with no nutritive value. Sometimes, ingredient listing can be misleading. When the word sugar is listed last, it can give the impression that the food has very little sugar. Actually, it can contain more sugar than is apparent. Other unfamiliar sugars may be in the food, but is listed in different names. Examples of other names for sugar are fruit juice, honey, invert sugar, lactose, and the like. These other terms for sugar can be interspersed with the other ingredients. For hidden sources or other names of sugar, salt, and fats, see page 195.

Food Standards

The FDA sets up food standards to avoid fraud and confusion to the consumer; and unfairness in competition. The absence of food standards would lead to the same food having different names or different foods having the same name. In the interest of consumers, the FDA is empowered by Section 401 of the Federal Food, Drug, and Cosmetic Act to establish regulations, as needed, for:

A reasonable definition and "standard of identity" – FDA defines what a specific product's name should be, and what ingredients must or maybe used in its manufacture. The exception to these are: butter, fresh and dried fruits and vegetables. However, standards of identity may be established for avocados, cantaloupes, citrus fruits, and melons.

A reasonable "standard of quality" – This is a minimum standard which establishes specifications for quality standards such as tenderness, color, and freedom from defects. Standards of quality have been set up for many vegetables. Foods not meeting these standards have to bear bold type labels which states:

"Below Standard in Quality"
"Good Food - Not High Grade"

It means that although it may be a wholesome food, yet it does not meet the usual expectations of the consumer. The quality standards are different from the standards for grades of meats and fish.

A reasonable "standard of fill-of-container" – These standards specify how full the container must be and how it is measured.

*"The existing fill-of-container standards for canned fruits and vegetables may be grouped as follows:

1. Those that require the maximum practicable quantity of the solid food that can be sealed in the container and processed by heat without crushing or breaking such component (limited to canned peaches, pears, apricots, and cherries).
2. Those requiring a minimum quantity of the solid food in the container after processing. The quantity is commonly expressed either as a minimum drained weight for a given container size or as a percentage of the water capacity of the container.
3. Those requiring that the food, including both solid and liquid packing medium, shall occupy not less than 90 percent of the total capacity of the container.

4. Those requiring both a minimum drained weight and the 90 percent minimum fill.

5. Those requiring a minimum volume of the solid component irrespective of the quantity of liquid (canned green peas and canned field peas). Fill-of-container standards specifying minimum net weight or minimum drained weight have been established for certain fish products....."

*(*An excerpt from Requirements of Laws and Regulations Enforced by the U.S. Food and Drug Administration, at:* –
http://www.fda.gov/opacom/morechoices/smallbusiness/blubook.htm)

Modified Foods

Traditional foods that have been modified, such as "reduced calorie" or "fat free" products, must follow these provisons:**

"1. Comply with the provisions of the standard for the traditional standardized food except for the deviation described by the nutrient content claim.

2. Not be nutritionally inferior to the traditional standardized food.

3. Possess performance characteristics, such as physical properties, flavor characteristics, functional properties, and shelf life, that are similar to those of the traditional standardized food, unless the label bears a statement informing the consumer of a significant difference in performance charactreristics that materially limits the use of the modified food (e.g., "not recommended for baking").

4. Contain a significant amount of any mandatory ingredient required to be present in the traditional standardized food.

5. Contain the same ingredients as permitted in the standard for the traditional standardized food, except that ingredients may be used to improve texture, prevent syneresis, add flavor, extend shelf life,

improve appearance, or add sweetness so that the modified food is not inferior in performance characteristics to the traditional standardized food...."

**(*An excerpt from Requirements of Laws and Regulations Enforced by the U.S. Food and Drug Administration, at http:// www.fda.gov/opa-com/morechoices/smallbusiness/blubook.htm*)

Imitation Foods

Imitation food resembles another food and is used as a substitute, but is nutritionally inferior to the food it imitates. It should bear in the label these words:

"Imitation (*name of food*)"

Exception to this rule, is when the quality of the substitute is equal or greater than the food imitated.

Genetically Engineered Foods

Genetically engineered foods are foods or crops whose genes have been artificially modified. Reasons for altering a vegetable or fruit's natural characteristic is to produce a crop resistant to pests, virus, or herbicides; or simply sidestep the traditional methods of breeding to produce a superior crop, for commercial reasons. The U.S. Government considers these foods as GRAS (generally recognized as safe) and does not require its labeling.

Consumer groups have already voiced their objections to these kind of foods. They fear that when these are sown or released in the field, it will not be possible to control cross pollination between species, thus promoting genetic pollution. This could result in an ecological imbalance as new resistant viruses or pests evolve. The consumer will end up as guinea pigs, since these foods have not been shown to be scientifically safe.

Different consumer groups are campaigning to pass a law requiring that these foods be properly labeled as such, so the buyer can make his own decision on the matter. These groups are also spreading information about the presence and impending growth of genetically engineered foods in the future markets. Those interested in knowing more about this agricultural bio-technology and its impact on our lives can go to Appendix A (private associations), page 221, for addresses. Below are some websites you can visit:

http://www.netlink.de/gen/home.html

http://www.emagazine.com/may-june-1998/0598feat2.html

http://www.biotechcentury.org/perils.html

Nutrient Content Descriptors

Nutrient content descriptors are terms such as "fat-free" or "high-fiber," used by manufacturers to describe the level of nutrients available in the product. No exact amount is mentioned, unlike "Nutrition Facts." Some nutrient content descriptors have many synonyms that signify the same thing or represent the same quality in the food. These synonyms are used interchangeably with the other nutrient content descriptors.

Nutrient Content Descriptors	Synonyms
Free	Without
	No
	Zero
	Trivial source of
	Dietarily insignificant source of
	Negligible source of
	Non (Non fat)
Low	Lo
	Little
	Few
	Low source of
	Contains a small amount of
Reduced	Fewer
	Lower in
	Less
High	Hi
	Rich in
	Excellent source
Light	Lite

Criteria for the use of Nutrient Content Descriptors

The following are the standards set by the FDA in order for food manufacters to use a nutrient claim in their food labels (for specific and exact numbers refer to www.fda.gov).

Criteria for the use of Nutrient Content Descriptors	
Free:	
➤ Calorie free	less than 5 calories
➤ Sodium free	less than 5 mg
➤ Sugar free	less than 0.5 g
➤ Fat free	less than 0.5 g
➤ Saturated fat free	less than 0.5 g, and not more than 1% of trans fatty acids from total fat
➤ Cholesterol free	less than 2 mg of cholesterol, and 2 g or less of saturated fat
➤ Percent (%) fat free	must be fat-free or low-fat, must reflect the amount present in 100 g of the food
Low:	
➤ Low calorie	40 calories or less
➤ Low sodium	140 mg or less
➤ Very low sodium	35 mg or less
➤ Low fat	3 g or less
➤ Low saturated fat	1 g or less
➤ Low cholesterol	20 mg or less and 2 g or less of saturated fat, if serving is 30 g or less, or 2 tbsps or less per 50 g of food
Reduced:	at least 25% less of a nutrient or 25% fewer calories than a reference* food
➤ Reduced cholesterol	at least 25% less and 2 g or less of saturated fat than a reference* food
High:	contains 20% or more of the Daily Value (DV) for a nutrient
➤ High fiber	5 g or more per serving, must be low fat or total fat stated beside high fiber claim
Good Source:	contains 10 to 19% of DV for a nutrient
➤ Good source of fiber	2.5 g to 4.9 g
More	at least 10% more of the DV than the reference* food
➤ Fortified, enriched, added	an altered food contains at least 10% more of the DV than the reference* food
➤ More or added fiber	at least 2.5 g or more than reference* food

Lean:	less than 10 g fat, 4.5 g or less saturated fat, and less than 95 mg cholesterol per 3.57 oz (100g) serving
➤ extra lean	less than 5 g fat, less than 2 g saturated fat, less than 95 mg cholesterol per 3.5 oz (100 g) serving
Healthy:	low in fat and saturated fat, containing no more than 360 mg (single item food and 480 mg (meal type) in sodium, and no more than 60 mg of cholesterol, plus:
	➤ if single item food – must provide at least 10% Daily Value of Vitamins A or C, iron, calcium, protein, or fiber
	➤ if meal type food – must provide 10% of 2 or 3 of the above-mentioned vitamins, minerals, proteins or fiber
Light – Lite:	food with 1/3 fewer calories or half the fat of the reference* food; if food derives 50% or more of its calories from fat, the reduction must be 50% of the fat
➤ light in sodium	a low calorie, low fat food with its sodium content reduced by at least 50%
➤ light meal	"low fat" or "low calorie" meal
➤ light	also used to describe texture and color such as "light brown sugar," or "light and fluffy"
Fresh:	food is raw, unprocessed, never frozen, never heated, and contains no preservatives; *exceptions:*
	➤ irradiation is allowed at low levels
	➤ "fresh milk"
	➤ "freshly baked bread"
Fresh Frozen:	frozen fresh – foods that are quickly frozen while still fresh; blanching or brief scalding is allowed to prevent nutrient breakdown
No Added Sugars:	without added sugar during processing or packing, including ingredients that in itself contains sugar; does not necessarily mean that it is low or reduced in calories
Low Calorie Meals:	120 calories or less per 100g

"Reference amounts" have been established by FDA for 139 different food product categories. These are food usually consumed per eating occasion by the average person.

Manufacturers are bound by FDA regulations to abide by the criteria set forth whenever they decide to use these terms. "Free," "Very Low," or "Low" can be used if the food meets the definition without benefit of special processing, alteration, formulation or reformulation.

General Descriptors and Statements in Food Packages

➤ **Product dates** – Descriptive words used before specific dates are:
   • *"Pull date"* or *"Sell by"* – last day for the product to be sold to remain fresh for home storage.
   • *"Packing date"* – date when food was manufactured, processed, or packaged.
   • *"Best if used by"* or *"Best before"* – These are not safety dates, but dates recommended for the food to be used, for optimal quality.
   • *"Expiry date"* – last day for food to be eaten. Usually these are used in perishable items, such as milk and eggs. After this date, freshness, palatability, or safety is not assured.
➤ **Religious Symbols** – Symbols of food prepared according to religious requirements, such as "Kosher" food prepared according to Jewish Dietary Laws, is not an FDA requirement. Some symbols are as follows:

Star-K   OU   OK   KOF-K

➤ **Grades, Standards and Inspection Symbols** – These are usually used for dairy products, meat, and orange juice. Grades and standards indicate quality in terms of texture, taste, and appearance, and do not suggest nutrient value. Inspection stamps on meat and poultry packages mean that the slaughter, processing, and packing of the meat meet the sanitary standards, as shown below:

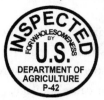

► **Universal Product Code** (UPC) – These black vertical bars with a 10-digit number identifies the manufacturer and product. It is used by the food industry for inventory control.

► **Trademarks and Copyrights** – "R" refers to a trademark for a brand name registered with the U.S. Patent and Trademark Office. "C" or "©" is indicative of a literary or artistic work protected under U.S. Copyright laws.

► **Safe Food Preparation, Handling, or Cooking Instructions** – Uncooked meat and poultry will contain instructions on how to prevent bacterial contamination. Some products that need cooking will suggest oven or microwave temperatures; and preparation, cooking, or serving tips. Heeding instructions will enable one to have safe and tastier food. An example is shown below.

STOVETOP DIRECTIONS
EMPTY contents carefully into medium skillet.
BRING just to a boil; drain, if desired.
Season to taste; serve.

MICROWAVE DIRECTIONS
EMPTY contents carefully into microwave-safe dish; cover.
MICROWAVE on HIGH for 2 1/2 to 3 1/2 minutes;
drain, if desired. Season to taste; serve.

► **"Natural," "pure," "health," "organic," "country"** – These terms do not necessarily equate with highly nutritious food. Read "Nutrition Facts" and "Ingredients" on food labels for assurance.

➤ **Homogenized** – Homogenization is the process of breaking up fat globules of milk into very fine particles, to give a smooth and uniform texture.

➤ **Pasteurized** – Pasteurization is the process of partial sterilization of a substance, such as milk or eggs. It needs a temperature high enough with a certain period of exposure, to destroy bacteria and inactivate enzymes that cause spoilage.

➤ **Ultra pasteurized** – This term is used for a food heated to a temperature higher than pasteurization to further extend shelf life of the food.

➤ **Ultra High Temperature** (UHT) – A term used when food is processed, comparable to ultra pasteurization, using high heat and sterilized containers. Food can be stored for three months without refrigeration, if unopened.

➤ **Enriched** – This means some nutrients lost during food processing are added to the finished product. Since not all lost nutrients are added, it is healthier to consume whole grains rather than enriched flour or enriched bread.

➤ **Fortified** – Fortification is adding nutrients to a food product that does not previously contain these nutrients in its original form. Check for high amounts of sugar or fats in the food labels. This may or may not be a healthy food.

Fat Descriptors for Milk

➤ 2% milk – "reduced" fat or "less" fat

➤ 1% milk – "low" fat or "little" fat

➤ skim milk – "fat-free," "zero fat," or "no fat" milk

Other Names for Sugar, Salt and Fats

➤ Other Names for Sugar

Sucrose (table sugar)
Beet sugar
Brown sugar
Cane sugar
Corn sweetener
Corn syrup
Dextrin
White sugar
Fruit juice
Galactose
Glucose
Glucose syrup

Lactose
Maltose
Maple sugar
Molasses
Sorbitol
Treacle/syrup
Turbinado sugar
Fructose
Honey
Hydolyzed starch
Invert sugar
Dextrose

➤Other Names for Salt

Sodium chloride (table salt)
Baking powder
Baking soda
Flavored salt
Self-rising flour
Any compound with "sodium:"
Anhydrous disodium phosphate
Sodium phosphate
Dioctyl sodium sulfosuccinate
Disodium dihydrogen pyrophosphate
Disodium guanylate
Disodium inosinate
Monosodium glutamate (MSG)
Sodium alginate
Sodium carboxymethyl cellulose
Sodium propionate
Sodium sulfite
Sodium citrate
Trisodium citrate
Sodium benzoate
Sodium caseinate
Sodium hydroxide
Sodium nitrite/nitrate

➤**Other Names for Saturated Fats**

Animal fats	Sour cream
Butter	Sweet cream
Coconut oil	Whole milk
Hydrogenated oil	Cheese
Palm oil	Shortening

Health Claims on Food Labels

At this time of writing, there are ten health claims allowed by FDA on food labels. These claims show a relationship between a food or nutrient, such as the reduction of a disease risk, or promotion of a health condition. These should be based on scientific evidence and used under certain conditions set by the FDA. This new FDA ruling is a great boon to the consumer as compared to the earlier practice of some manufacturers who made misleading and inaccurate claims. These health claims should make the consumer realize the importance of nutrition in promoting health. Hereunder are the authorized health claims:

1. Calcium and Osteoporosis

Osteoporosis is a condition marked by bone porosity and fragility that can easily lead to skeletal weakness and fractures. In terms of nutrition, a regular and adequate intake of calcium can reduce the risk of osteoporosis later in life. Aside from nutrition, an added factor that can help prevent this condition is regular progressive resistance and weight-bearing exercises.

2. Sodium and Hypertension

Hypertension or high blood pressure can be a harbinger for heart attack or stroke. A diet low in sodium (salt) is one way to reduce the risk of high blood pressure.

3. Fats and Cancer

Cancers of the breast, colon, and prostate are linked to high fat diets, not discounting other genetic and external factors. A diet low in fat (less than 30% of total daily caloric allowance) may reduce the risk of fat-related cancers.

4. Saturated fat/Cholesterol and Coronary Heart Disease (CHD)

A combination of saturated fat and cholesterol leads to high blood cholesterol, and eventually to CHD. In terms of dietary guidelines, reduce the risk of CHD by:

➤ decreasing saturated fat intake to less than 10% of total daily caloric allowance; and
➤ decreasing daily cholesterol intake to less than 300 mg.

5. Fiber and Cancer

Grains, fruits, and vegetables are the usual sources of dietary fiber. Fiber absorbs fats and toxins, and excretes these substances expeditiously. These are probably the reasons why dietary fiber in the diet may reduce the risk of some cancers.

6. Fruits/Vegetables and Cancer

Fruits and vegetables contain fiber and are usually low in fat, reducing the risk of cancer. In addition, phytochemicals and nutrients in plant foods such as Vitamin C, antioxidants, beta-carotene, and polyphenols, may prevent cancer and promote resistance to diseases.

7. Soluble Fiber and Coronary Heart Disease

Soluble fibers bind with fats and cholesterol, thus lowering the amounts absorbed by the body into its system. Soluble fibers that come from grain, fruits, and vegetables can reduce the risk of coronary heart disease, when included in the regular diet.

8. Folate and Neural Tube Birth Defects

Neural tube birth defects such as *spina bifida* are development defects of the spinal cord and spinal nerves of the fetus. A child born with such a defect can have symptoms like clubfoot, hydrocephalus, hip dislocation, curvature of the spine (*scoliosis*), loss of kidney function, muscle weakness, and spasm. Since neural tube defects occur within the first six weeks of conception, a woman planning to become pregnant should already include an adequate amount of folate (folic acid) in her diet. This may reduce the risk of having a child with neural tube birth defects.

9. Sugar and Dental Cavities

It is common knowledge that sugar (sucrose) contributes to tooth decay and dental cavities. According to FDA, there are some sugar alcohols that do not promote tooth decay, such as xylitol, sorbitol, mannitol, and maltitol.

10. Whole Oats/Psyllium Seed Husk and Coronary Heart Disease

Whole oats and psyllium seed husks are two soluble fibers authorized by FDA to be used in the claim of manufacturers, that these foods can reduce the risk of coronary heart disease.

These health claims are optional, and not all manufacturers avail of them. In the future, we will probably have more allowable health claims approved by the FDA.

SURVIVAL IN THE FOOD JUNGLE

Chapter 10

Compromises and Adjustments

Everyone wants to have a balanced diet or a weight-loss diet that works. Busy schedules, lack of information and planning – all waylay a person from one's objectives. The keeping of high fat and sugary foods in the refrigerator make one an easy prey for temptation. In order to eat healthy foods, they need to be accessible in the food pantry or kitchen. This makes it helpful and easier to stick to a healthy diet.

In the real world, it is only practical to make compromises and adjustments. An occasion may arise where one finds oneself eating unsafe or "forbidden foods." All is not lost, when this happens. One can always make up for it by making sure that the next meals are healthy ones, to make up for this lapse.

Foods we find delicious are mostly those we are used to or those that we have eaten since childhood. Taste is a matter of habit. Strange foods from different cultures may be distasteful to us. Yet, these other cultures may also find our own food unappetizing, bland, weird, or too spicy – depending on which part of the world we originate.

There are more delicious and healthier foods out there, waiting for you to discover. Let your taste buds thrill to new flavors and savor the adventure in world cuisine. Try the different food pyramids or make your own.

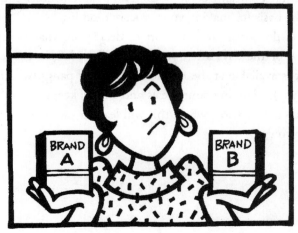

Substitutes for High-Fat Foods

Substitute	High-Fat Foods
Chicken & turkey breast,lean meat, fish	Marbled red meats
Microwaved, baked, broiled, roast, boiled, poached, steamed foods	Fried foods
Non-fat milk, skim milk, 1% fat milk	Whole milk
Low-fat or non-fat salad dressings (mayonnaise and sour creams) low-fat yogurt, or cheese	High-fat salad dressings, yogurt, & cheese
Jam, jelly, fruit preserves, low-fat butter, whipped butter	Butter
Soft margarine, hummus	Stick margarine
Angel food cake, baked or dried fruits, low-fat cookies, fresh fruits, low-fat cakes	Butter cakes, other regular cakes, cookies, & pastries
Air-popped popcorn, low-fat chips, rice cakes, oatmeal cookies`	Regular chips, crackers

Meal Planning
List of Meals and Snacks

Before venturing out to the grocery store or supermarket for a week or so of food supplies, write down the meals that you want to prepare. Include also the snacks. If new to this undertaking, consult some low-fat or health cookbooks. The planned meals and snacks will be the basis for making your grocery food list.

If you do not make the effort to decide on what foods to eat tomorrow or the days after, your diet will be left to chance or to whatever is available at the moment of hunger pangs (whatever the food maybe). Planning your meals and snacks keeps you in control of your diet. You know where this will lead to - more savings and a healthier you!

Grocery List of Health Foods to Choose from:

➤ *Fruits:*

Cantaloupe	Mango
Grapefruit	Avocado
Oranges	Peaches
Strawberries	Cherries
Apples	Nectarine
Papaya	Grapes
Banana	Prunes
Apricots	

➤ *Vegetables:*

Dry Beans	Asparagus
Carrots	Pumpkin
Broccoli	Mushrooms
Kale/Collard	Artichoke
Fresh Beans	Cauliflower
Brussel Sprouts	Cabbage
Bell/Chilli Peppers	Onions/Tomatoes

➤ *Carbohydrates/Fiber:*

Whole Wheat Flour	Whole Grain Bread
Whole Grain Cereal	Whole Wheat Pasta
Egg Pasta	Oats
Potatoes	Brown Rice
Corn Tortilla	Sweet Potato

➤ *Fats:*

Almonds	Sunflower Seeds/Oil
Pumpkin Seeds	Safflower Oil
Olive Oil	Flaxseed
Canola Oil	

➤ *Protein:*

Fish	Tofu
Lean Meat	Eggs
Skim Milk	Cottage Cheese
Chicken/Turkey Breast	Nonfat Yogurt
Chicken Drumsticks	Skim Milk

➤ *Spices/Condiments/Seasonings:*

Garlic	Blackstrap Molasses
Ginger	Honey
Ground pepper	Organic Soy Sauce
Cilantro	Apple Cider Vinegar
Ground Cayenne	Oregano
Brown Sugar	Bay leaf
Curry Powder	Tomato Sauce
Paprika	Ketchup
Salt	Basil

Your Own Food List

Make your own grocery list of what foods to buy. This food list you come up with, will facilitate decision-making when you are at the supermarket. It will not only save you time and money, but promote health for you and your family. On the basis of your planned meals and snacks, make a list of foods or ingredients you intend to buy. Refer to "Health Foods and Diet Choices", Chapter 8. You will also find the simplified "grocery list of health foods to choose from" and "substitutes for high-fat foods" in the preceding pages, greatly helpful.

Food Shopping Guide

Your food list can complement or augment the "Food Shopping Guide" shown in the next pages. Both your food list and shopping guide can be a handy reminder to bring to the supermarket when making purchases. The food shopping guide contains:

➤ A list of additives to avoid
➤ Reminder for allergies or medical problems
➤ A suggested list of healthy foods

There are two shopping guides to choose from:

Shopping Guide No.1. – It has all of the above-mentioned contents
Shopping Guide No.2 – It has a list of the harmful additives only, and you fill in the rest of the blank area. Customize it to suit your planned meals, your pyramid, or healthy food choices.

"Reminder" (Found below back of Shopping Guides):

If you or a family member is allergic to an additive or food, write down this person's name and the substance he is allergic to. Under "Health Notes," write down whatever important health matter or medical problem you need to be reminded of, like: *Sodium – not more than 1,000 mg,"* or *"No red meat,"* or *"Buy only organic milk,"* and the like. The shopping guide of your choice will be a handy reference when you go shopping for food. As soon as you are aware of another additive considered harmful, add it to your shopping guide list in the "AVOID" section.

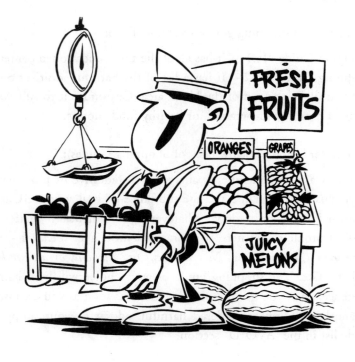

FOOD SHOPPING GUIDE #1

AVOID

- Acesulfame K
- Cyclamate
- Nitrites
- Potassium Bromate
- Irradiated Foods
- Hydrogenated Vegetable Oil
- BHA/BHT/TBHQ
- Aluminum
- Red No. 40 (Allura AC)
- Red No.3 (Erythrosine)
- Blue No. 2 (Indigotine)
- Citrus Red No.2
- Cochineal (Carminic Acid)

- Aspartame
- Saccharin
- Sulfites
- Brominated Vegetable Oil
- BGH/BST Hormone
- MSG/HVP
- Olestra
- Quinine
- Yellow No. 5 (Tartrazine)
- Blue No. 1 (Brilliant Blue)
- Green No. 3 (Fast Green)
- Yellow No. 6 (Sunset Yellow)

FOODS TO BUY

Fruits:

- Cantaloupe
- Grapefruit
- Oranges
- Strawberries
- Apples
- Papaya
- Banana
- Avocado

- Mango
- Apricots
- Peaches
- Cherries
- Nectarine
- Grapes
- Prunes

Vegetables:

- Spinach
- Carrots
- Broccoli
- Kale
- Fresh Beans
- Cauliflower
- Cabbage
- Okra

- Asparagus
- Pumpkin
- Mushrooms
- Onions/Tomatoes
- Dry Beans
- Brussel Sprouts
- Bell/Chilli Peppers
- Collard

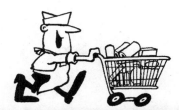

FOOD SHOPPING GUIDE #1

Carbohydrates/Fiber:

- Whole Wheat Flour
- Whole Grain Cereal
- Egg Pasta
- Potatoes
- Corn Tortilla
- Whole Grain Bread
- Whole Wheat Pasta
- Oats
- Brown Rice
- Sweet Potato

Fats:

- Almonds
- Olive Oil
- Sunflower Seeds/Oil
- Flaxseed
- Pumpkin Seeds
- Canola Oil
- Safflower Oil

Proteins:

- Fish
- Chicken/Turkey Breast
- Tofu
- Cottage Cheese
- Skim Milk
- Lean Meat
- Chicken Drumsticks
- Eggs
- Nonfat Yogurt

Spices/Condiments/Seasonings:

- Ginger
- Salt
- Ground Cayenne
- Honey
- Curry Powder
- Apple Cider Vinegar
- Bay Leaf
- Ketchup
- Cilantro
- Basil
- Garlic
- Ground Pepper
- Brown Sugar
- Blackstrap Molasses
- Organic Soy Sauce
- Oregano
- Tomato Sauce
- Paprika

Reminder:

Allergic to: Person's Name:

_____   _____
_____   _____
                                                 _____

Health Notes

_____
_____

FOOD SHOPPING GUIDE #2

AVOID

- Acesulfame K
- Cyclamate
- Nitrites
- Potassium Bromate
- Irradiated Foods
- Hydrogenated Vegetable Oil
- BHA/BHT/TBHQ
- Aluminum
- Red No. 40 (Allura AC)
- Red No.3 (Erythrosine)
- Blue No. 2 (Indigotine)
- Citrus Red No.2
- Cochineal (Carminic Acid)

- Aspartame
- Saccharin
- Sulfites
- Brominated Vegetable Oil
- BGH/BST Hormone
- MSG/HVP
- Olestra
- Quinine
- Yellow No. 5 (Tartrazine)
- Blue No. 1 (Brilliant Blue)
- Green No. 3 (Fast Green)
- Yellow No. 6 (Sunset Yellow)

FOODS TO BUY

Fruits:

Vegetables:

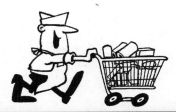

Carbohydrates/Fiber:

Fats:

Proteins:

Spices/Condiments/Seasonings:

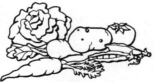

Reminder:

Allergic to: Person's Name:

_____   _____

_____   _____

_____   _____

Health Notes

_____

_____

From Supermarket to Kitchen

Buying at the Supermarket

➤ Shop first in the outside lanes where fresh foods are kept.

➤ Shop last in the frozen foods area.

➤ Do not buy gray-colored, funny smelling, or discolored meat.

➤ Put meat in another plastic bag.

➤ Do not buy opened, dented, and out-of-shape cans or packages.

➤ Given a choice, buy food in a bottle or glass container rather than in a can or carton.

➤ Buy locally produced vegetables and fruits, especially those in season.

Watch Out for Taste Enhancers

If you are watching your salt, fat, or sugar intake, read the labels. Some low fat foods may contain more salt than expected. Or some low sodium foods may contain high amounts of fat. Some non-fat, and sodium-free foods may contain large amounts of sugar.

Handling and Preparing Food

➤ Wash hands before and after touching food.

➤ Wash all fruits and vegetables before using them.

➤ Follow instructions on food packages, such as:
  • Do not thaw until ready for use
  • Refrigerate after opening
  • Keep in cool dry place

➤ When defrosting meat or fish, put in a larger tray to catch thawed liquid.

➤ Wipe fluids that drop or seep out from thawed foods with disposable kitchen towels.

➤ Paper towels are preferable over cloth towels. Throw away used paper towels.

➤ Do not eat foods containing uncooked eggs.

➤ Left-over canned goods should be transferred to non-metallic covered containers in the freezer.

➤ Avoid re-thawing of one product several times. When buying a big amount of seafood, fish, or meat, rewrap these in smaller portions before putting them in the freezer.

➤ Use 2 cutting boards – one for meat and one for vegetables. Otherwise, clean cutting boards thoroughly before subsequent use.

➤ Trim fat from meat.

➤ Do not wash fresh fish and seafood before freezing to preserve freshness and flavor.

➤ Thaw and clean fish and seafood only when it will be cooked right away.

➤ Cook fish and seafood before it is thoroughly thawed.

➤ Do not refreeze thawed fish and seafood.

Cooking

➤ Prefer steaming over boiling, to retain more nutrients.

➤ Do not put too much water when boiling food, unless you want to make soup.

➤ Cook meat thoroughly.

➤ Boil water first before dropping the fish or vegetables into the pot.

➤ For pots and pans use glass, stainless steel, or cast iron, rather than aluminum.

➤ Use teflon-coated pans to lessen the use of cooking oil.

➤ Cooked meat broth can be placed in the refrigerator (let it cool off first) so fat can be removed when it solidifies.

➤ To kill harmful bacteria, observe the right cooking (internal) temperature in order to cook food thoroughly. You will need a cooking thermometer, which can be bought at the local supermarket.

Correct Cooking Temperatures	
RAW FOOD **Ground Products**	**INTERNAL** **TEMPERATURE**
Hamburger	160°F
Beef, veal, lamb, pork	160°F
Chicken, turkey	165°F
Beef, Veal, Lamb Roasts & Steaks	
Medium-rare	145°F
Medium	160°F
Well-done	170°F
Pork Chops, roast, ribs	
Medium	160°F
Well-done	170°F
Ham, fresh	160°F
Sausage, fresh	160°F
Poultry Chicken, whole & pieces	
Duck	
Turkey *(unstuffed)*	180°F
Whole	180°F
Breast	170°F
Dark meat	180°F
Stuffing (cooked separately)	165°F
Eggs Fried, poached	Yolk & white are firm
Casseroles	160°F
Sauces, custards	160°F

The preceding chart has been adapted for home use and is consistent with consumers guidelines from the U.S. Department of Agriculture (USDA) and the U.S. Food & Drug Administration (FDA).

Food Supply Problems

The food supply in the United States is one of the safest in the world. Yet, a lot of work still need to be done to minimize the exposure of consumers to food hazards. Problems, described below, need timely solutions before they become unwieldy:

➤ Consumers are trying to eat more fruits and vegetables, some of which come from other countries that do not have high safety standards of food inspection. Even some of our local produce are contaminated with traces of pesticides.

➤ Our "nine to five" working people are relying more and more on counter take-outs, prepared, frozen and restaurant foods, for themselves and their families. How will the authorities adequately monitor businesses who are preparing these kinds of foods?

➤ Changes in food consumption patterns and fast-paced developments in food production, processing, and marketing can lead to disarray.

➤ Microorganisms are developing resistance to some control agents and antibiotics.

➤ Recalls of contaminated food have led consumers to question the trust accorded to the food producers and the food safety monitoring authorities. Annually, an estimate of 9,000 deaths and 6.5 to 33 million illnesses are attributed to food hazards.

➤ Information on food additives and safety in food shopping gets to the consumers in bits and dribbles, and sometimes in vague and confusing terms. These are usually not readily available to the average consumer.

➤ Some research and studies are based on political and economic convenience, and what a few may falsely assume as the common "good."

➤ After careful research and studies, authorities and scientists dealing with food production and regulations find it difficult to implement changes on food safety measures. This is due to public apathy in embracing innovations due to fear (founded or otherwise) of health consequences.

Role of Consumer in Food Safety

More Consumer Awareness

Since the Food, Drug and Cosmetic Act in 1938 was passed, several amendments, regulations, and memoranda of agreement, related hereto, were enacted. After 60 years, several federal agencies have been established to promote the mandate of the Food, Drug and Cosmetic Act. Most consumers are not aware of the existence of these agencies and the role they play. Most issues are placed at the doorstep of the Food and Drug Administration (FDA). Consumers do not know the numerous work and great responsibilities entailed in providing them safe foods. Activities like research and education, collection of data, monitoring, surveillance, inspection, enforcement and outbreak management (plus consumer service and administrative duties) – involve a lot of supporting budget, manpower, and authority.

Federal Agencies Involved in Food Safety

➤ Agricultural Marketing Service
➤ Animal and Plant Health Inspection Service
➤ Agricultural Research Service
➤ Cooperative State Research
➤ Education and Extension Service
➤ Food Safety and Inspection Service
➤ Grain Inspection, Packers and Stockyards Administration of the USDA
➤ Centers for Disease Control and Prevention
➤ Food and Drug Administration
➤ National Institutes of Health of the Department of Health and Human Services
➤ National Marine Fisheries Service of the Department of Commerce
➤ Environmental Protection Agency

The existence of the above agencies would appear to necessitate a coordinator or a coordinating system. Without a coordinator to oversee all the different functions of these many agencies, there is bound to be a duplication of work and the neglect of some important activities. If a coordinating system is not possible, the FDA should be given more power and resources to enable it to do the job they need to perform.

Consumer Power

Most consumers fold their arms nonchalantly and abide by the notion that only federal institutions are responsible for the public's food health and safety. Consumers do not realize that there is a necessity to take direct responsibility for their own health by investing a little time and effort on their part toward the following:

➤ Inform relevant institutions of problems, concerns, and interests about food consumption so that appropriate actions are taken accordingly.

➤ Inform manufacturers and grocery stores if a product is damaged or harmful. Refusing to buy this kind of product will send a message to the manufacturers to stop producing it.

➤ Do not be misled by ridiculous food advertisement and sales pitch.

➤ Keep abreast of factual news, research results, and new programs of government relating to food.

➤ Those interested in consumer group action can get information through the internet, magazines, or the library.

Inspite of the dangers lurking in the the jungle, it can still be an oasis. As long as you know where the dangers and pitfalls are, you can avoid them and enjoy good health. This book can be your source of constant reference and also serve as a launching pad for seeking other useful information which will serve as guides to your survival in the food jungle.

Appendix **A**

Organizations and Information Sources*

Government:

United States Department of Agriculture (USDA)
Center for Nutrition Policy and Promotion
14th & Independence Ave., SW, Suite 240-E
Washington, D.C. 20250
http://www. usda. gov

FSIS Food Safety Education and Communications Staff
Room 1175, South Building
1400 Independence Ave., SW
Washington, D.C. 20250
Meat & Poultry Hotline: 1-800-535-4555
http://www.fsis.usda.gov
http://www.nalusda.gov

Food and Drug Administration (FDA)

➤ **Freedom of Information Office**
   Room 12-A-16, Parklawn Building
   5600 Fishers Lane, Rockville, MD 20857
   (301) 443-18   1-800-532-4440

➤ **FDA Consumer Food Information line**
   200 C St. S.W., HFS-555
   Washington, DC 2020
   Food Information & Seafood Hotline: 1-800-332-4010
   http://www.fda.gov

Environmental Protection Agency
401 M Street, SW
Washington, D.C. 20460
(202) 260-2090
http://www.epa.gov

Office of Ground Water and Drinking Water (4601)
401 M Street, SW
Washington, D.C. 20460-0003
(202) 260-5543
Safe Drinking Water Hotline: 1-800-426-4791
http://www.epa.gov/safewater/about.html

National Health Information Center (NHIC)
US Dept. of Health & Human Services
P.O. Box 1133, Washington, D.C. 20013-1133
(301) 565-4167   Fax: (301) 984-4256
Health Information Resources: 1-800-336-4797
email: nhicinfo@health.org
http://nhic-nt.health.org

National Cholesterol Education Program
Information Center
P.O. Box 30105
Bethesda, MD 20824-0105
(301) 251-1222
http://www.nhlbi.nih.gov/nhlbi/

National Cancer Institute
Cancer Information service:
1-800-422-6237
http://www.nci.nih.gov

Medical & Health Associations:

American Cancer Society
1599 Clifton Road
Atlanta, GA 30329
1-800-ACS-2345

American Dietetic Association
216 W. Jackson Boulevard, Suite 800
Chicago, IL 60606-6995
(For a Registered Dietitian in Your Area): 1-800-366-1655
(312) 899-0040   http://www.eatright.org

American Heart Association
National Center
7272 Greenville Ave.
Dallas, TX 75231
(Customer Heart & Stroke Information): 1-800-242-8721
(Women's Health Information): 1-800-MY-HEART
Health Questions:
http://www.americanheart.org/email/INQemail.html

American Medical Association

➤ *Headquarters:*
    515 North State Street
    Chicago, IL 60610
      (312) 464-5000

➤ *Washington Office:*
    1101 Vermont Ave., NW
    Washington, D.C. 20005
      (202) 789-7400
      http://www.ama.assn.org/

Private Associations:

American Institute for Cancer Research
P.O. Box 97167
Washington, D.C. 20090-7167
(202)328-7744   1-800-843-8114

Campaign For Food Safety
(formerly Pure Food Campaign)
860 Highway 61, Little Marais, MN 55614
(218) 226-4164   Fax: (218) 226-4157
email: alliance@mr.net   http://www.purefood.org

Center for Science in the Public Interest (CSPI)
1875 Connecticut Ave. NW, Ste.300
Washington, D.C. 20009
(202) 332-9110
Fax:(202) 265-4954   email: cspi@cspinet.org
http://www.cspinet.org

Feingold Association of the United States
127 E. Main Street #106
Riverhead, NY 11901
(516) 369-9340   Fax (516) 369-2988
http://www.fiengold.org   (a not-for-profit organization
educating the public as to the relationship of behavior, learning and
health, to food and food additives; more specifically with Attention
Deficit Disorder (AD/HD), Pervasive Developmental Delays
(PDD), autism and salicylate sensitivities.)

NoMSG
P.O. Box 367
Santa Fe, NM 87504
(800) 232-8674   email: info@nomsg.com

S.T.O.P. (Safe Tables Our Priority)
P.O. Box 46522
Chicago, IL 60646-0522
(312) 957-0284   Fax (312) 427-2307

Water Quality Association
4151 Naperville Road
Lisle, IL 60532
(708) 505-0160

Food and Water
RR1 Box 68D
Walden, VT 05873
1-800-EAT-SAFE

Alliance for Bio-Integrity
P.O. Box 110
Iowa City, IA 52244-0110
(515) 472-5554   Fax: (515) 472-6431
email: infor@bio-integrity.org   http://www.bio-integrity.org

The Campaign (to Label Genetically Engineered Foods)
P.O. Box 55699
Seattle, WA 98155
(425) 771-4049   http://www.thecampaign.org

Consumer Right to Know/Safety First
P.O. Box 1177
Fairfield, IA 52556
(515) 472-2809   Hotline: (877) REAL-FOOD
http://www.safe-food.org

Not an exclusive listing

BGH/BST-Free Dairy Producers*

Alta Dena Certified Dairy
17637 E. Valley Blvd.
City of Industry, CA 91744
(626) 964-6401
For a Store Location Near You: 1-800-MILK-123
http://www.altadenadairy.com

Ben & Jerry's Homemade Holdings, Inc.
30 Community Drive
South Burlington, VT 05403-6828
(802) 846-150   email: package@benjerry.com
http://www.benjerry.com

Hartzler Family Dairy, Inc.
5454 Cleveland Road (Rt. 3)
Wooster, OH
(330) 345-8190
http://www.hartzler.eyemg.cm

Horizon Organic Dairy, Inc.
P.O. Box 17577
Boulder, CO 80308-7577
email: info@horizonorganic.com

Newman's Own Ice Cream Partnership
30 Community Drive
So. Burlington, VT 05403-6828

Organic Valley/CROPP Cooperative
507 W. Main St.
La Farge, WI 54639
(608) 625-2602   Fax: (608) 625-2600
http://www.organicvalley.com

Promised Land Dairy
Rt 3 Box 197C
Floresville, TX 78114
(830) 216-4200

Stonyfield Farm
10 Burton Drive
Londonderry, NH 03053
(603) 437-5050   http://www.stonyfield.com

Joseph Farms
10561 West Highway 140
P.O. Box 775
Atwater, CA 95301
(209) 394-7984   Fax (209) 394-4988
email: info@josephfarms.com
Http://josephfarmscheese.com/hormone.shtm

Not an exclusive listing

Food Producers Not Using Pesticides, Antibiotics, Hormones*

Meat Products:

Laura's Lean Beef Company
2285 Executive Dr., Ste. 200
Lexington, KY 40505
1-800-ITS-LEAN
http://www.laurasleanbeef.com

North Hollow Farms
RR1, Box 47
Rochester, VT 05767
(802) 767-4255   email: nhollow@sover.net
http://www.naturalmeat.com

Roseland Organic Farms
27427 M-60 West
Cassopolis, MI 49031
(616) 445-8769   Fax: (616) 445-8987
email: macmerrill@aol.com (also supplies organic cheese, dairy
products, other produce)

Walnut Acres Organic Farms
Walnut Acres Road
Penns Creek, PA 17862
1-800-433-3998   email: customerservice@walnutacres.com
http://www.walnutacres.com (also supplies baked goods, cereals,
other produce)

Other Organic Products:

Horizon Organic Dairy, Inc.
P.O. Box 17577,
Boulder, Co 80308-7577
1-888-494-3020   email: webmaster@horizonorganic.com
http://www.horizonorganic.com (fruit juice, butter, sour cream, yogurt, other dairy products)

Cascadian Farm, Inc.
Rockport, WA 98283
27427 M-60 West
1-800-624-4123   http://www.cfarm.com
email: consumerservice@smallplanetfoods.com
(fruit juice, frozen vegetables & fruits, prepared meals)

Lundberg Family Farms
5370 Church Street
Post Office Box 369
Richvale, CA 95974-0369
(530) 882-4551   Fax: (530) 882-450
http://www.lundberg.com
(organic rice variieties)

Unbromated Bread and Flour Products:

Nature's Own
Flowers Bakeries, Inc
Thomasville, GA 31757

Pepperidge Farm, Inc.
General Office
Norwalk, CT 06856

Not an exclusive listing

Appendix **D**

How to Report Adverse Reactions and Other Problems with Products Regulated by FDA

January 1, 1999

Consumers can play an important public health role by reporting to the U.S. Food and Drug Administration any adverse reactions or other problems with products the agency regulates. FDA is responsible for ensuring that foods are safe, wholesome, and correctly labeled. It also oversees medicines, medical devices (from bandages to artificial hearts), blood products, vaccines, cosmetics, veterinary drugs, animal feed, and electronic products that emit radiation (such as microwave ovens and video monitors), ensuring that these products are safe and effective.

The testing that helps to establish the safety of products, such as drugs and medical devices, is typically conducted on small groups before FDA approves the products for sale. Some problems can remain unknown, only to be discovered when a product is used by a large number of people.

When problems with FDA-regulated products occur, the agency wants to know about them and has several ways for the public to make reports. Timely reporting by consumers, health professionals, and FDA-regulated companies allows the agency to take prompt action. The agency evaluates each report to determine how serious the problem is, and, if necessary, may request additional information from the person who filed the report before taking action.

Reporting an Emergency

If the situation is an emergency that requires immediate action, such as a case of food-borne illness or a drug product that has been tampered with, call the agency's main emergency number, staffed 24 hours a day, 301-443-1240.

You also can report emergencies to an FDA consumer complaint coordinator in your geographic area. *A list of all the coordinators' phone numbers* is provided in this document.

Non-Emergency Reports

If you experience a problem that does not require immediate action – such as a non-emergency adverse reaction to a food product or an over-the-counter medical device that doesn't work as advertised – you can report it to the appropriate Consumer Complaint Coordinator listed on page 2 (*page 230 of this book*). Or you can report it to the appropriate FDA office from the following list:

Foods

➤ To report problems, including adverse reactions, related to any food except meat and poultry, contact the district office consumer complaint coordinator for your geographic area. A list of all the coordinators' phone numbers is provided.

➤ If the problem involves meat or poultry, which are regulated by the U.S. Department of Agriculture, call the USDA hotline at 1-800-535-4555.

Medicines (prescription and over-the-counter), medical devices, blood products and other biologicals, special nutritional products (dietary supplements, infant formula, medical foods)

FDA's MedWatch program is designed for health professional and consumer reporting of serious adverse events and problems with medical products, so that these events and problems can be monitored. An adverse event is considered serious if the outcome attributed to the event is: death; a life-threatening situation; admission to a hospital or a longer-than-expected hospital stay; permanent disability; a birth defect; or medical/surgical care to prevent permanent impairment or damage.

In addition, MedWatch works to ensure that new safety information is quickly communicated to the health professional community. The program aims to enhance postmarketing surveillance of medical products as they are used in clinical practice, so that FDA can, as rapidly as possible, identify serious reactions and hazards associated with these products. To report a problem to MedWatch:

➤ If you or a family member has experienced or witnessed a serious adverse event or other problem with a medical product, you can obtain a MedWatch form by:

➤ Calling MedWatch at 1-800-FDA-1088 (1-800-332-1088) to request that a reporting form (one-page, return postage paid) and instructions on how to complete the form be mailed to you.

➤ Downloading a form and instructions from the MedWatch Website at *http://www.fda.gov/medwatch/how.htm.* Completed forms can be mailed to FDA at the address on the back of the form or faxed to 1-800-FDA-0178 (1-800-332-0178).

➤ You can also report directly to FDA by using the interactive form available on the MedWatch Website at *http://www.accessdata.fda.gov/medwatch/medwatch-online.htm.*

➤ FDA encourages consumers to take the form to their health professional (doctor, dentist, pharmacist, or nurse) to complete. This person can provide much more detailed clinical information, such as laboratory results, which can help FDA evaluate the report. Since reporting by health professionals is voluntary, consumers are encouraged to file a report on their own if they prefer that a health professional not fill out the form or if the health professional chooses not to report the problem.

➤ FDA also welcomes reports through MedWatch of product quality problems. For example, you can report product contamination (suspicious foul odors or unusual "off" colors); defective components; labeling concerns (such as mix-ups due to similar names or packaging); or questionable product stability.

Vaccines

Adverse reactions and other problems related to vaccines should be reported to the Vaccine Adverse Event Reporting System, which is maintained by FDA and the Centers for Disease Control and Prevention. For a copy of the vaccine reporting form, call 1-800-822-7967 or on the FDA website at *http://www.fda.gov/cber/vaers.html.*

Veterinary Products

Report any problems with veterinary drugs and animal feed to FDA's Center for Veterinary Medicine at 1-888-FDA-VETS (1-888-332-8387).

Cosmetics

Call the FDA Cosmetics and Colors Automated Information Line 1-800-270-8869, for information on how to report adverse reactions to cosmetics, as well as problems such as filth, decomposition, or spoilage.

Medical Advertising

To report fraudulent or misleading advertising or promotion of FDA-regulated products, call 1-800-238-7332.

General Guidelines About Reporting

➤ Report what happened as soon as possible. Give names, addresses and phone numbers of persons affected. Include your name, address and phone number, as well as that of the doctor or hospital if emergency treatment was provided.

➤ State the problem clearly. Describe the product as completely as possible, including any codes or identifying marks on the label or container. Give the name and address of the store where the product was purchased and the date of purchase.

➤ You also should report the problem to the manufacturer or distributor shown on the label and to the store where you purchased the product.

What FDA Doesn't Handle

Reports and complaints about the following should be made to the agencies listed. Phone numbers can be found in your local phone directory:

➤ Restaurant food and sanitation – Local or state health departments

➤ Unsolicited products in the mail – U.S. Postal Service

➤ Accidental poisonings – Poison control centers or hospitals

➤ Pesticides or air and water pollution – U.S. Environmental Protection Agency

➤ Hazardous household products (including toys, appliances, and chemicals) – Consumer Product Safety Commission, 1-800-638-2772

➤ Alcoholic beverages – Department of Treasury's Bureau of Alcohol, Tobacco and Firearms

➤ Drug abuse and controlled substances – Department of Justice's Drug Enforcement Administration

➤ Hazardous chemicals in the workplace – Department of Labor's Occupational Safety and Health Administration

➤ Warranties – Federal Trade Commission

➤ Dispensing and sales practices of pharmacies – State board of pharmacy

➤ Medical practice – State certification board

General Information

If you have a general question about an FDA-regulated product, call 1-800-532-4440. But please don't report problem products or adverse reactions to this consumer information number. Use the other numbers described above.

FDA's Consumer Complaint Coordinators

To report adverse reactions or other problems with FDA-regulated products, contact the FDA district office consumer complaint coordinator for your geographic area:

Alabama – (615) 781-5385, ext. 123
Alaska – (425) 483-4949
Arizona – (714) 798-7701
Arkansas – (214) 655-5310, ext. 521
California (Northern) – (510) 337-6741
California (Southern) – (714) 798-7701

Colorado – (303) 236-3044
Connecticut – (781) 279-1675, ext. 188
Delaware – (215) 597-9064
District of Columbia – (410) 962-3593
Florida (Northern) – (407) 475-4717
Florida (Southern) – (305) 526-2800, ext. 916
Georgia – (404) 347-4001, ext. 5272
Hawaii – (510) 337-6741
Idaho – (425) 483-4949
Illinois – (312) 353-7840
Indiana – (313) 226-6260, ext. 171
Iowa – (913) 752-2440
Kansas – (913) 752-2440
Kentucky – 1-800-437-2382
Louisiana – (504) 589-7186, ext. 150
Maine – (781) 279-1675, ext. 188
Maryland – (410) 962-3593
Massachusetts – (781) 279-1675, ext. 188
Michigan – (313) 226-6260, ext. 171
Minnesota – (612) 334-4100, ext. 184
Mississippi – (504) 589-7186, ext. 150
Missouri – (913) 752-2440
Montana – (425) 483-4949
Nebraska – (913) 752-2440
Nevada – (510) 337-6741
New Hampshire – (781) 279-1675, ext. 188
New Jersey – (973) 331-2917
New Mexico – (303) 236-3044
New York (Northern) – (716) 551-4461, ext. 3171
New York (Southern) – (718) 340-7000, ext. 5725
North Carolina – (404) 347-4001, ext. 5272
North Dakota – (612) 334-4100, ext. 184
Ohio – 1-800-437-2382
Oklahoma – (214) 655-5310, ext. 521

Oregon – (425) 483-4949
Pennsylvania – (215) 597-9064
Rhode Island – (781) 279-1675, ext. 188
South Carolina – (404) 347-4001, ext. 5272
South Dakota – (612) 334-4100, ext. 184
Tennessee – (615) 781-5385, ext. 123
Texas – (214) 655-5310, ext. 521
Utah – (303) 236-3044
Vermont – (781) 279-1675, ext. 188
Virginia – (410) 962-3593
Washington – (425) 483-4949
West Virginia – (410) 962-3593
Wisconsin – (612) 334-4100, ext. 184
Wyoming – (303) 236-3044
Puerto Rico, U.S. Virgin Islands – (787) 729-6728

This backgrounder replaces "Reporting Problems with FDA-Regulated Products," BG 91.9.1 (November 1991), BG 98-3 (April 1998), and BG 98-5 (August 1998)
(BG 99-1)

This is a mirror of the page at http://www.fda.gov/opacom/back-grounders/problem.html

Onset, Duration, and Symptoms of Foodborne Illness*

Approximate Onset Time to Symptoms After Eating/Exposure	Predominant Symptoms	Associated Organism or Toxin
Upper gastrointestinal tract symptoms (nausea, vomiting) occur first or predominate		
Less than 1 h	Nausea, vomiting, unusual taste, burning of mouth	Metallic salts
1-2 h	Nausea, vomiting, cyanosis, headache, dizziness, dyspnea, trembling, weakness, loss of consciousness	Nitrites
1-6 h mean 2-4 h	Nausea, vomiting, retching, diarrhea, abdominal pain, prostration	*Staphylococcus aureus* and its entero-toxins
8-16 h (2-4 h emesis possible)	Vomiting, abdominal cramps, diarrhea, nausea	*Bacillus cereus*
6-24 h	Nausea, vomiting, diarrhea, thirst, dilation of pupils, collapse, coma	Amanita species mushrooms

Sore throat and respiratory symptoms occur

12-72 h	Sore throat, fever, nausea, vomiting, rhinorrhea (free discharge of thin nasal mucus), sometimes a rash	*Streptococcus pyogenes*
2-5 days	Inflamed throat and nose, spreading grayish exudate, fever, chills, sore throat, malaise, difficulty in swallowing, edema of cervical lymph node	*Corynebacterium diphtheriae*

Lower gastrointestinal tract symptoms (abdominal cramps, diarrhea) occur first or predominate

2-36 h, mean 6-12 h	Abdominal cramps, diarrhea, putrefactive diarrhea associated with *C. perfringens*, sometimes nausea and vomiting	*Clostridium perfringens, Bacillus cereus, Streptococcus faecalis, S. faecium*
12-74 h, mean 18-36 h	Abdominal cramps, diarrhea, vomiting, fever, chills, malaise, nausea, headache - possible. Sometimes bloody or mucoid diarrhea, cutaneous lesions associated with *V. vulnificus*. *Yersinia enterocolitica* mimics flu and acute appendicits	*Salmonella* species (including *S. arizonae*), *Shigella*, entero-pathogenic *Escherichia coli*, other Enterobacteriacae, *Vibrio parahaemolyticus, Yersinia enterocolitica, Pseudomonas aeruginosa* (?), *Aeromonas hydrophila, Plesiomonas shigelloides, Campylobacter jejuni, Vibrio cholerae* (O1 and non-O1) *V. vulnificus, V. fluvialis*

3-5 days	Diarrhea, fever, vomiting, abdominal pain, resspiratory symptoms	Enteric viruses
1-6 weeks	Mucoid diarrhea (fatty stools), abdominal pain, weight loss.	*Giardia lamblia*
1 to several weeks	Abdominal pain, diarrhea, constipation, headache, drowsiness, ulcers, variable - often asymptomatic.	*Entamoeba histolytica*
3-6 months	Nervousness, insomnia, hunger pains, anorexia, weight loss, abdominal pain, sometimes gastroenteritis	*Taenia saginata, T. solium*
Neurological symptoms (visual disturbances, vertigo, tingling, paralysis) occur		
Less than 1 h	*** SEE GASTROINTESTINAL AND/OR NEUROLOGIC SYMPTOMS (Shellfish Toxins) - (page 239)	Shellfish toxin
	Gastroenteritis, nervousness, blurred vision, chest pain, cyanosis, twitching, convulsions	Organic phosphate
	Excessive salivation, perspiration, gastroenteritis, irregular pulse, pupils constricted, asthmatic breathing	Muscaria-type mushrooms
	Tingling and numbness, dizziness, pallor, gastrohemmorrhage, and desquamation of skin, fixed eyes, loss of reflexes, twitching, paralysis	Tetradon (tetrodotoxin) toxins

1-6 h	Tingling and numbness, gastroenteritis, dizziness, dry mouth, muscular aches, dilateded pupils, blurred vision, paralysis	Ciguatera toxin
	Nausea, vomiting, tingling, dizziness, weakness, anorexia, weight loss, confusion	Chlorinated hydrocarbons
2 h to 6 day usually 12-36 h	Vertigo, double or blurred vision, loss of reflex to light, difficulty in swallowing, speaking, and breathing, dry mouth, weakness, respiratory paralysis	*Clostridium botulinum* and its neurotoxins
More than 72 h	Numbness, weakness of legs, spastic paralysis, impairment of vision, blindness, coma	Organic mercury
	Gastroenteritis, leg pain, ungainly high-stepping gait, foot and wrist drop	Triorthocresyl phosphate
Allergic symptoms (facial flushing, itching) occur		
Less than 1 h	Headache, dizziness, nausea, vomiting, peppery taste, burning of throat, facial swelling and flushing, stomach pain, itching of skin	Histamine (scombroid)
	Numbness around mouth, tingling sensation, dizziness, headache, nausea	Monosodium glutamate

	Flushing, sensation of warmth, itching, abdominal pain, puffing of face and knees	Nicotinic acid

Generalized infection symptoms (fewer, chills, malaise, prostration, aches, swollen lymph nodes) occur

4-28 days, mean 9 days	Gastroenteritis, fever, edema about eyes, perspiration muscular pain, chills, prostration, labored breathing	*Trichinella spiralis*
7-28 days, mean 14 days	Malaise, headache, fever, cough, nausea, vomiting, constipation, abdominal pain, chills, rose spots, bloody stools	*Salmonella typhi*
10-13 days	Fever, headache, myalgia, rash	*Toxoplasma gondii*
10- 50 days, mean 25-30 days	Fever, malaise, lassitude, anorexia, nausea, abdominal pain, jaundice	Etiological agent not yet isolated - probably viral
Varying periods (depends on specific illness)	Fever, chills, head- or joint ache, prostration, malaise, swollen lymph nodes, and other specific symptoms of disease in question	*Bacillus anthracis, Brucella melitensis, B. abortus, B. suis, Coxiella burnetii, Francisella tularensis, Listeria monocytogenes, Mycobacterium tuberculosis, Mycobacterium species, Pasteurella multocida, Streptobacillus moniliformis, Campylobacter jejuni, Leptospira species.*

Gastrointestinal and/or Neurologic Symptoms - (Shellfish Toxins)

0.5 to 2 hr	Tingling, burning, numbness, drowsiness, incoherent speech, respiratory paralysis	Paralytic Shellfish Poisoning (PSP) (saxitoxins)
2-5 min to 3-4 h	Reversal of hot and cold sensation, tingling; numbness of lips, tongue & throat; muscle aches, dizziness, diarrhea, vomiting	Neurotoxic Shellfish Poisoning (NSP) (brevetoxins)
30 min to 2-3 h	Nausea, vomiting, diarrhea, abdominal pain, chills, fever	Diarrheic Shellfish Poisoning (DSP) (dinophysis toxin, okadaic acid, pectenotoxin, yessotoxin)
24 h (gastrointestinal) to 48 h (neurologic)	Vomiting, diarrhea, abdominal pain, confusion, memory loss, disorientation, seizure, coma	Amnesic Shellfish Poisoning (ASP) (domoic acid)

*Adapted from: Bad Bug Book - Foodborne Pathogenic Microorganisms and Natural Toxins Handbook. U.S. Food & Drug Administration/Center for Food Safety and Applied Nutrition.

Food Product Recalls (January-August, 1999)

➤ Firm Recalls Cooked Sausage for Possible *Listeria* Contamination (August 27, 1999)

➤ Puerto Rico Firm Recalls Chorizos for Potential *Salmonella* and *Listeria* (August 26, 1999)

➤ Baltimore Firm Recalls Sausage for Possible *Salmonella* (August 18, 1999)

➤ New Hampshire Company Recalls Beef Patties for Potentially Harmful *E. coli* O157 contamination (August 6, 1999)

➤ Pennsylvania Firm Recalls Hot Dogs for Possible *Listeria* Contamination (July 30, 1999)

➤ New Jersey Firm Recalls Sausage for Possible *Listeria* Contamination (July 30, 1999)

➤ Michigan Firm Recalls Sliced Hams for Possible *Listeria* Contamination (July 29, 1999)

➤ Texas Company Recalls Beef Tips in Gravy Because of Undercooking (July 16, 1999)

➤ Sausages Recalled in Hawaii Because of *Listeria monocytogenes* (June 18, 1999)

➤ Chicken Nuggets Recalled for Undeclared Whey (June 15, 1999)

➤ North Dakota Meat Company Recalls Wieners for *Listeria* Contamination (June 1, 1999)

➤ Pennsylvania Meat Company Recalls Weisswurst Sausage for *Listeria* Contamination (May 28, 1999)

➤ North Carolina Firm Recalls Luncheon Meats for Potential *Listeria* Contamination (May 14, 1999)

➤ Utah Firm Recalls Ham With Potential *Salmonella* (May 13, 1999)

➤ USDA Declares Product from Thorn Apple Valley's Forrest City, Arkansas Plant Unfit for Human Consumption (April 13, 1999)

➤ New York Grocery Recalls Ground Beef Contaminated With *E.. coli* O157:H7 (April 13, 1999)

➤ New Jersey Firm Recalls Franks (Mark 18, 1999)

➤ Los Angeles Firm Recalls Egg Rolls for Undeclared Egg Whites (March 2, 1999)

➤ California Firm Recalls Egg Rolls Because of Undeclared Egg Whites (February 25, 1999)

➤ Georgia Firm Recalls Franks and Smoked Sausages for *Listeria* (February 18, 1999)

➤ Chicago Meat Company Recalls Headcheese for *Listeria* (February 17, 1999)

➤ Washington State Meat Company Recalls Hot Dogs for *Listeria* Contamination (February 5, 1999)

➤ Ontario Meat Company Recalls Cooked Sausage for *Listeria* Contamination (February 5, 1999)

➤ Bil Mar *Listeria* Recall - Additional Brands Sold at Retail (January 28, 1999)

➤ Thorn Apple Valley *Listeria* Recall - Update and Amended List (January 28, 1999)

➤ Thorn Apple Valley Frankfurters and Lunch Combination Products Recalled for Potential *Listeria* Contamination (January 22, 1999)

➤ Ohio Meat Company Recalls Deli Meat for *Listeria* (January 22, 1999)

➤ Oscar Mayer Recalls Deli Meat for *Listeria* (January 15, 1999)

Adapted from: http://www.fsis.usda. gov/OA/news/xrecalls.htm

Appendix **G**

HOW SMOKING CONTRIBUTES TO CARDIOVASCULAR DISEASES AND OTHER AILMENTS

The nicotine and carbon monoxide, in cigarettes and cigarette smoke, respectively, are two substances that contribute to cardiovascular disease:

Nicotine – Nicotine constricts blood vessels which can increase blood pressure. It induces the formation of blood clots which can cause heart attacks. Nicotine triggers the release of adrenalin which, in turn, causes the heart to pump faster and harder. This action can be life threatening if the coronary arteries are already blocked. Excess adrenalin can also lead to heartbeat irregularities.

Carbon Monoxide – Carbon monoxide is a dangerous substance found in cigarette smoke. It reduces the amount of oxygen by 20%, thereby reducing its needed availability in the body system. The released adrenalin increases the heart's need for oxygen, while the carbon monoxide reduces the amount of oxygen. Smokers who are not aware of their having blood clots are candidates for heart attacks and strokes.

Other dangers of smoking are: lung cancer, cancer of the lip and other parts of the respiratory system, cancer of the urinary bladder, chronic bronchitis, and emphysema. These diseases, among others, are caused by the carcinogens and toxic substances in the cigarette smoke. The saliva that contains these substances irritates the body tissues that it comes in contact with, causing corrosive damage. This makes the tissues easily susceptible to cancer and other diseases, since it is unable to perform its normal functions.

Appendix **H**

Blood Lipid Levels:

➤ Total Cholesterol
➤ Triglycerides
➤ High Density Lipoproteins
➤ Low Density Lipoproteins

Total Blood Cholesterol Levels

Levels		mg/dl
Desirable	less than	200
Borderline High		200-239
High		240 or more

Blood Triglyceride Levels

Levels		mg/dl
Normal	less than	200
Borderline High		200 to 400
High		400 to 1000
Very High		Over 1000

Triglyceride measurements are taken after fasting from food and alcohol overnight (12 hours).

HDL and LDL Desirable Levels

Levels		mg/dl
HDL		35 or higher
LDL	less than	130

Recommended Dietary Allowances (RDA) for Adults

Vitamin/ Mineral	NM*	Male	Female	Age (years)
A	mcg RE	1000	800	15-51+
D	mcg	10	10	15-24
		5	5	25-51+
E	mg a-TE	10	8	15-51+
K	mcg	65	55	15-18
		70	60	19-24
		80	65	25-51+
C	mg	60	60	15-51+
Thiamin	mg	1.5	1.1	15-50
		1.2	1.0	51+
Riboflavin	mg	1.8	1.3	15-18
		1.7	1.3	19-50
		1.4	1.2	51+
Niacin	mg NE	20	15	15-18
		19	15	19-50
		15	15	51+
B-6 mg	2.0	1.5		15-18
		2.0	1.6	19-51+
Folate	mcg	200	180	15-51+
B-12	mcg	2.0	2.0	15-51+
Calcium	mg	1200	1200	15-14
		800	800	25-51+
Phosphorus	mg	1200	1200	15-24

		800	800	25-51+
Magnesium	mg	400	300	15-18
		350	280	19-51+
Iron	mg	12	15	15-18
		10	15	19-50
		10	10	51+
Zinc	mg	15	12	15-51+
Iodine	mcg	150	150	15-51+
Selenium	mcg	50	50	15-18
		70	55	19-51+

Adapted from the USDA "Recommended Dietary Allowances (RDA)"

For children's RDA and other details, visit :
http://www..nal.usda.gov/fnic/Dietary/chartis.gif
in the internet.

*Nutrient Measures (NM)

➤ **g** (grams) – equivalent to 0.03 ounces
➤ **mg** (milligrams) – one thousandth of a gram
➤ **mcg** (micrograms) – one millionth of a gram
➤ **mg NE** (milligrams niacin equivalents) – a measure of niacin activity
➤ **mg a-TE** (milligrams alpha tocopherol equivalents) – a measure of Vitamin E activity
➤ **mcg RE** (micrograms retinol equivalents) – a measure of Vitamin A activity

Current Drinking Water Standards*

National Primary and Secondary Drinking Water Regulations

I. National **Primary** Drinking Water Regulations (NPDWRs or primary standards) are legally enforceable standards that apply to public water systems. Primary standards protect drinking water quality by limiting the levels of specific contaminants that can adversely affect public health and are known or anticipated to occur in public water systems.

II. National **Secondary** Drinking Water Regulations (NSDWRs or secondary standards) are non-enforceable guidelines regulating contaminants that may cause cosmetic effects (such as skin or tooth discoloration) or aesthetic effects (such as taste, odor, or color) in drinking water. EPA recommends secondary standards to water systems but does not require systems to comply. However, states may choose to adopt them as enforceable standards.

Contaminant Levels

MCLG (Maximum Contaminant Level Goal) – The maximum level of a contaminant in drinking water at which no known or anticipated adverse effect on the health effect of persons would occur, and which allows for an adequate margin of safety. MCLG's are *non-enforceable* public health goals.

MCL (Maximum Contaminant Level) – The maximum permissible level of a contaminant in water which is delivered to any user of a public water system. MCLs are *enforceable* standards. The margins of safety in MCLGs ensure that exceeding the MCL slightly does not pose significant risk to public health.

TT(Treatment Technique) – An *enforceable* procedure or level of technical performance which public water systems must follow to ensure control of a contaminant.

Water contaminants are divided into:

A. Inorganic chemicals
B. Organic chemicals
C. Radionuclides
D. Microorganisms

I. NATIONAL PRIMARY DRINKING WATER REGULATIONS

Contaminants	MCLG (mg/l)*	MCL or TT (mg/l)*
	Contaminant Levels:	

A. *INORGANIC CHEMICALS:*

➤ **Antimony**   0.006   0.006
Potential Health Effects:: Increase in blood cholesterol; decrease in blood glucose
Sources: Discharge from petroeum refineries; fire retardants; ceramics; electronics; solder

➤ **Arsenic:**   none[1]   0.05
Potential Health Effects: Skin damage; circulatory system problems; increased risk of cancer
Sources: Discharge from semiconductor manufacturing; petroleum refining; wood preservatives; animal feed additives; herbicides; erosion of natural deposits

➤ **Asbestos**   7 million   7 MFL
(fiber > 10 micrometers)   fibers per
                                            liter(MFL)
Potential Health Effects: Increased risk of developing benign intestinal polyps
Sources: Decay of asbestos cement in water mains; erosion of natural deposits

➤ **Barium**   2   2
Potential Health Effects: Increase in Blood pressure
Sources: Discharge of drilling wastes; discharge from metal refineries; erosion of natural deposits

➤ **Beryllium**   0.004   0.004
Potential Health Effects: Intestinal lesions
Sources: Discharge from metal refineries and coal-burning factories; discharge from electrical, aerospace, and defense industries

➤ **Cadmium**   0.005   0.005
Potential Health Effects: Kidney damage
Sources: Corrosion of galvanized pipes; erosion of natural deposits; discharge from metal refineries; runoff from waste batteries and paints

➤ **Chromium** (total)   0.1   0.1
Potential Health Effects: Some people who use water containing chromium well in excess of the MCL over many years could experience allergic dermatitis
Sources: Discharge from steel and pulp mills; erosion of natural deposits

➤ **Copper**   1.3   <u>Action</u>
                                             <u>Level=1.3;</u>
                                             <u>TT</u>[2]

Potential Health Effects: **Short term exposure:** Gastrointestinal distress. **Long term exposure:** Liver or kidney damage. Those with Wilson's Disease should consult their personal doctor if their water systems exceed the copper action level.
Sources: Corrosion of household plumbing systems; erosion of natural deposits; leaching from wood preservatives

➤ **Cyanide** (as free cyanide)   <u>0.2</u>   <u>0.2</u>
Potential Health Effects: Nerve damage or thyroid problems
Sources: Dischaarge from steel/metal factories; discharge from plastic and fertilizer factories

➤**Fluoride**   4.0   4.0
Potential Health Effects: Bone disease (pain and tenderness of the bones); children may get mottled teeth
Sources: Water additive which promotes strong teeth; erosion of natural deposits; discharge from fertilizer and aluminum factories

➤ **Lead**   <u>zero</u>   <u>Action</u>
                                             <u>Level=0.015;</u>
                                             <u>TT</u>[2]

Potential Effects: Infants and children: Delays in physical or mental development. Adults: Kidney problems; high blood pressure
Sources: Corrosion of household plumbing systems; erosion of natural deposits

➤ **Inorganic Mercury**   <u>0.002</u>   <u>0.002</u>
Potential Health Effects: Kidney damage
Sources: Erosion of natural deposits; discharge from refineries and factories; runoff from landfills and cropland

➤ **Nitrate** (measured   10   10
as Nitrogen)
Nitrite (measured   1   1
as Nitrogen)

Potential Health Effects: "Blue baby syndrome" in infants under six months – life threatening without immediate medical attention. Symptoms: Infant looks blue and has shortness of breath.
Sources: Runoff from fertilizer use; leaching from septic tanks, sewage; erosion of natural deposits

➤ **Selenium**   0.05   0.05

Potential Health Effects: Hair or fingernail loss; numbness in fingers or toes; circulatory problems
Sources: Discharge from petroleum refineries; erosion of natural deposits; discharge from mines

➤ **Thalium**   0.0005   0.002

Potential Health Effects: Hair loss; changes in blood; kidney, intestine, or liver problems
Sources: Leaching from ore-processing sites; discharge from electronics, glass, and pharmaceutical companies

B. *ORGANIC CHEMICALS*

➤ **Acrylamide**   zero   TT[3]

Potential Health Effects: Nervous system or blood problems; increased risk of cancer
Sources: Added to water during sewage/wastewater treatment

➤ **Alachlor**   zero   0.002

Potential Health Effects: Eye, liver, kidney or spleen problems; anemia; increased risk of cancer
Sources: Runoff from herbicide used on row crops

➤ **Atrazine** <u>0.003</u> <u>0.003</u>
Potential Health Effects: Cardiovascular system problems; reproductive difficulties
Sources: Runoff from herbicide used on row crops

➤ **Benzene** <u>zero</u> <u>0.005</u>
Potential Health Effects: Anemia; decrease in blood platelets; increased risk of cancer
Sources: Discharge from factories; leaching from gas storage tanks and landfills

➤ **Benzo(a)pyrene** <u>zero</u> <u>0.0002</u>
Potential Health Effects: Reproductive difficulties; increased risk of cancer
Sources: Leaching from linings of water storage tanks and distribution lines

➤ **Carbofuran** <u>0.04</u> <u>0.04</u>
Potential Health Effects: Problems with blood or nervous system; reproductive difficulties
Sources: Leaching of soil fumigant used on rice and alfalfa

➤ **Carbon tetrachloride** zero .005
Potential Health Effects: Liver problems; increased risk of cancer
Sources: Discharge from chemical plants and other industrial activities

➤ **Chlordane** <u>zero</u> <u>0.002</u>
Potential Health Effects: Liver or nervous system problems; increased risk of cancer
Sources: Residue of banned termiticide

➤ **Chlorobenzene**   <u>0.1</u>   <u>0.1</u>
Potential Health Effects: Liver or kidney problems
Sources: Discharge from chemical and agricultural chemical factories

➤ **2,4-D**   <u>0.07</u>   <u>0.07</u>
Potential Health Effects: Kidney, liver, or adrenal gland problems
Sources: Runoff from herbicide used on row crops

➤ **Dalapon**   <u>0.2</u>   <u>0.2</u>
Potential Health Effects: Minor kidney changes
Sources: Runoff from herbicide used on rights of way

➤ **1,2-Dibromo-3-**   <u>zero</u>   <u>0.0002</u>
  chloropropane (DBCP)
Potential Health Effects: Reproductive difficulties; increased risk of cancer
Sources: Runoff/leaching from soil fumigant used on soybeans, cotton, pineapples, and orchards

➤ **o-Dichlorobenzene**   <u>0.6</u>   <u>0.6</u>
Potential Health Effects: Liver, kidney, or circulatory system problems
Sources: Discharge from industrial chemical factories

➤ **p-Dichlorobenzene**   <u>0.075</u>   <u>0.075</u>
Potential Health Effects: Anemia; liver, kidney or spleen damage; changes in blood
Sources: Discharge from industrial chemical factories

➤ **1,2-Dichloroethane**   <u>zero</u>   <u>0.005</u>
Potential Health Effects: Increased risk of cancer
Sources: Discharge from industrial chemical factories

➤ **1-1-Dichloroethylene**   0.007   0.007
Potential Health Effects: Liver problems
Sources: Discharge from industrial chemical factories

➤ **cis-1,2-Dichloro-**   0.07   0.07
  ethylene
Potential Health Effects: Liver problems
Sources: Discharge from industrial chemical factories

➤ **trans-1,2-Dichloro-**   -   0.1   0.1
  ethylene
Potential Health Effects: Liver problems
Sources: Discharge from industrial chemical factories

➤ **Dichloromethane**   zero   0.005
Potential Health Effects: Liver problems; increased risk of cancer
Sources: Discharge from pharmaceutical and chemical factories

➤ **1-2-Dichloropropane**   zero   0.005
Potential Health Effects: Increased risk of cancer
Sources: Discharge from industrial chemical factories

➤ **Di(2-ethylhexyl)**   0.4   0.4
  adipate
Potential Health Effects: General toxic effects or reproductive difficulties
Sources: Leaching from PVC plumbing systems; discharge from chemical factories

➤ **Di(2-ethylhexyl)**   zero   0.006
  phthalate
Potential Health Effects: Reproductive difficulties; liver problems; increased risk of cancer
Sources: Discharge from rubber and chemical factories

➤ **Dinoseb**   0.007   0.007
Potential Health Effects: Reproductive difficulties
Sources: Runoff from herbicide used on soybeans and vegetables

➤ **Dioxin (2,3,7,8-TCDD)**   zero   0.00000003
Potential Health Effects: Reproductive difficulties; increased risk of cancer
Sources: Emissions from waste incineration and other combustion; discharge from chemical factories

➤ **Diquat**   0.02   0.02
Potential Health Effects: Cataracts
Sources: Runoff from herbicide use

➤ **Endothall**   0.1   0.1
Potential Health Effects: Stomach and intestinal problems
Sources: Runoff from herbicide use

➤ **Endrin**   0.002   0.002
Potential Health Effects: Nervous system effects
Sources: Residue of banned insecticide

➤ **Epichlorohydrin**   zero   TT[3]
Potential Health Effects: Stomach problems; reproductive difficulties; increased risk of cancer
Sources: Discharge from industrial chemical factories; added to water during treatment process

➤ **Ethylbenzene**   0.7   0.7
Potential Health Effects: Liver or kidney problems
Sources: Discharge from petroleum refineries

➤ **Ethelyne dibromide**   zero   0.00005
Potential Health Effects: Stomach problems; reproductive difficulties; increased risk of cancer
Sources: Discharge from petroleum refineries

➤ **Glyphosate**   0.7   0.7
Potential Health Effects: Kidney problems; reproductive difficulties
Sources: Runoff from herbicide use

➤ **Heptachlor**   zero   0.0004
Potential Health Effects: Liver damage; increased risk of cancer
Sources: Residue of banned termiticide

➤ **Heptachlor epoxide**   zero   0.0002
Potential Health Effects: Liver damage; increased risk of cancer
Sources: Breakdown of heptachlor

➤ **Hexachlorobenzene**   zero   0.001
Potential Health Effects: Liver or kidney problems; reproductive difficulties; increased risk of cancer
Sources:: Discharge from metal refineries and agricultural chemical factories

➤ **Hexachlorocyclo-**   0.05   0.05
     pentadiene
Potential Health Effects: Kidney or stomach problems
Sources: Discharge from chemical factories

➤ **Lindane**   0.0002   0.0002
Potential Health Effects: Liver or kidney problems
Sources: Runoff/leaching from insecticide used on cattle, lumber, gardens

➤ **Methoxychlor**   0.04   0.04
Potential Health Effects: Reproductive difficulties
Sources: Runoff/leaching from insecticide used on fruits, vegetables, alfalfa, livestock

➤ **Oxamyl (Vydate)**   0.2   0.2
Potential Health Effects: Slight nervous system effects
Sources: Runoff/leaching from insecticide used on apples, potatoes, and tomatoes

➤ **Polychlorinated**   zero   0.0005
  biphenyls (PCBs)
Potential Health Effects: Skin changes; thymus gland problems; immune deficiencies; reproductive or nervous system difficulties; increased risk of cancer
Sources: Runoff from landfills; discharge of waste chemicals

➤ **Pentachlorophenol**   zero   0.001
Potential Health Effects: Liver or kidney problems; increased risk of cancer
Sources: Discharge from wood preserving factories

➤ **Picloram**   0.5   0.5
Potential Health Effects: Liver problems
Sources: Herbicide runoff

➤ **Simazine**   0.004   0.004
Potential Health Effects: Problems with blood
Sources: Herbicide runoff

➤ **Styrene**   0.1   0.1
Potential Health Effects: Liver, kidney, and circulatory problems
Sources: Discharge from rubber and plastic factories; leaching from landfills

➤ **Tetrachloroethylene**   <u>zero</u>   <u>0.005</u>
Potential Health Effects: Liver problems; increased risk of cancer
Sources: Leaching from PVC pipes; discharge from factories and dry cleaners

➤ **Toluene**   <u>1</u>   <u>1</u>
Potential Health Effects: Nervous system, kidney, or liver problems
Sources: Discharge from petroleum factories

➤ **Total Trihalome-**   <u>none</u>[1]   <u>0.10</u>
   thanes (TTHMs)
Potential Health Effects: Liver, kidney or central nervous system problems; increased risk of cancer
Sources: Byproduct of drinking water disinfection

➤ **Toxaphene**   <u>zero</u>   <u>0.003</u>
Potential Health Effects: Kidney, liver, or thyroid problems; increased risk of cancer
Sources: Runoff/leaching from insecticide used on cotton and cattle

➤ **2,4,5-TP (Silvex)**   <u>0.05</u>   <u>0.05</u>
Potential Health Effects: Liver problems
Sources: Residue of banned herbicide

1,2,4-Trichlorobenzene   <u>0.07</u>   <u>0.07</u>
Potential Health Effects: Changes in adrenal glands
Sources: Discharge from textile finishing factories

➤ **1,1,1-Trichloroethane**   <u>0.20</u>   <u>0.2</u>
Potential Health Effects: Liver, nervous system, or circulatory problems
Sources: Discharge from metal degreasing sites and other factories

➤ 1,1,2-Trichloroethane   <u>0.003</u>   <u>0.005</u>
Potential Health Effects: Liver, kidney, or immune system problems
Sources: Discharge from industrial chemical factories

➤ Trichloroethylene   <u>zero</u>   <u>0.005</u>
Potential Health Effects: Liver problems; increased risk of cancer
Sources: Discharge from petroleum refineries

➤ Vinyl chloride   <u>zero</u>   <u>0.002</u>
Potential Health Effects: Increased risk of cancer
Sources: Leaching from PVC pipes; discharge from plastic factories

➤ Xylenes (total)   <u>10</u>   <u>10</u>
Potential Health Effects: Nervous system damage
Sources: Discharge from petroleum factories; discharge from chemical factories

C. *RADIONUCLIDES*

➤ **Beta particles and**   none[1]   <u>4 millirems</u>
photon emitters   <u>per year</u>
Potential Health Effects: Increased risk of cancer
Sources: Decay of natural and man-made deposits

➤ **Gross alpha particle**   none[1]   <u>15 picocuries</u>
activity   <u>per Liter</u>
                                                    <u>(pCi/L)</u>
Potential Health Effects: Increased risk of cancer
Sources: Erosion of natural deposits

➤ **Radium 226 and**   none[1]   <u>5 pCi/L</u>
Radium 228 (combined)
Potential Health Effects: Increased risk of cancer
Sources: Erosion of natural deposits

D. *MICROORGANISMS:*

➤ *Giardia lamblia*   zero   TT[4]
Potential Health Effects: Giardiasis, a gastroenteric disease
Sources: Human and animal fecal waste

➤ **Heterotrophic**   N/A   TT[4]
plate count
Potential Health Effects: HPC has no health effects, but can indicate
how effective treatment is at controlling microorganisms
Sources: n/a

➤ *Legionella*   zero   TT[4]
Potential Health Effects: Legionnaire's Disease, commonly known as
pneumonia
Sources: Found naturally in water, multiplies in heating systems

➤ **Total Coliforms**   zero   5.0%[5]
(including fecal coliform and *E. Coli)*
Potential Health Effects: Used as an indicator that other potentially
harmful bacteria may be present[6]
Sources: Human and animal fecal waste

➤ **Turbidity**   N/A   TT[4]
Potential Health Effects: Turbidity has no health effects but can interfere with disinfection and provide a medium for microbial growth. It
may indicate the presence of microbes.
Sources: Soil runoff

➤ **Viruses (enteric)**   zero   TT[4]
Potential Health Effects: Gastroenteric disease
Sources: Human and fecal waste

*Units are in milligrams per Liter (mg/L) unless otherwise noted.

[1]MCLGs were not established before the 1986 Amendments to the Safe Drinking Water Act. Therefore, there is no MCLG for this contaminant.

[2]Lead and copper are regulated in a Treatment Technique which requires systems to take tap water samples at sites with lead pipes or copper pipes that have lead solder and/or are served by lead service lines. The action level, which triggers water systems into taking treatment steps if exceeded in more than 10% of tap water samples, for copper is 1.3 mg/L, and for lead is 0.015 mg/L.

[3]Each water system must certify, in writing, to the state (using third-party or manufacturer's certification) that when acrylamide and epichlorohydrin are used in drinking water systems, the combination (or product) of dose and monomer level does not exceed the levels specified, as follows:

➤ **Acrylamide** = 0.05% dosed at 1 mg/L (or equivalent)
➤ **Epichlorohydrin** = 0.01% dosed at 20 mg/L (or equivalent)

[4]The Surface Water Treatment Rule requires systems using water or ground water under the direct influence of surface water to (1) disinfect their water, and (2) filter their water to meet criteria for avoiding filtration so that the following contaminants are controlled at the following levels:

➤ *Giardia lamblia:* 99.9% killed/inactivaated
➤ Viruses: 99.99% killed/inactivated
➤ *Legionella:* No limit, but EPA believes that if *Giardia* and viruses are inactivated, *Legionella* will also be controlled.
➤ Turbidity: At no time can turbidity (cloudiness of water) go above 5 nephelolometric turbidity units (NTU); systems that filter must ensure that the turbidity go no higher than 1 NTU (0.5 NTU for conventional or direct filtration) in at least 95% of the daily samples for any two consecutive months.
➤ HPC: No more than 500 bacterial colonies per milliliter.

[5]No more than 5.0% samples total coliform-positive in a month. (For water systems that collect fewer than 40 routine samples per month, no more than one sample can be total coliform-positive). Every sample that has total coliforms must be analyzed for fecal coliforms. There cannot be any fecal coliforms.

[6]Fecal coliform and *E. coli* are bacteria whose presence indicates that the water may be contaminated with human and animal wastes. Microbes in these wastes can cause diarrhea, cramps, nausea, headaches, or other symptoms.

II. NATIONAL SECONDARY DRINKING WATER REGULATIONS

Contaminant	Secondary Standard Contaminant Levels
Aluminum	0.05 to 0.2 mg/L
Chloride	250 mg/L
Color	15 (color units)
Copper	1.0 mg/L
Corrosivity	non-corrosive
Fluoride	2.0 mg/L
Foaming Agents	0.5 mg/L
Iron	0.3 mg/L
Manganese	0.05 mg/L
Odor	3 threshold odor number
pH	6.5-8.5
Silver	0.10 mg/L
Sulfate	250 mg/L
Total Dissolved Solids	500 mg/L
Zinc	5 mg/L

--------------------------------*Adapted from "Current Drinking Water Standards" of the Office of Ground Water and Drinking Water (OGWDW), United States Environmental Protection Agency (EPA). Revised September 21, 1998. (*To see the original document, visit the internet at: http://www.epa.gov/OGWDW/wot/appa.html).

Appendix **K**

Calculate Your Daily Caloric Allowance

Data needed: Gender
                      Weight
                      Age
                      Activity Level

A. First, find out your basal metabolic rate (BMR):
Male: weight X 12 = **BMR**
Female :   weight X 11 = **BMR**

B. Second, find out your age-adjusted BMR:
   For 30 -year Old and Over

Age Level	% of Age Level
30 to 39	2% (use .02)
40 to 49	4% (use .04)
50 to 59	6% (use .06)
60 to 69	8% (use .08)
70 to 79	10% (use .10)

BMR X (% of Age Level) = Age Factor;
BMR MINUS Age factor = **Age-Adjusted BMR**

C. Lastly, get your daily caloric allowance (DCA):
   Activity level

Description	Level	%
Sedentary	Very Light	10% (use .10)
Housework	Light	15% (use .15)
Calisthenics	Moderate	20% (use .20)
Aerobics	Heavy	30% (use. 30)
Athletics	Very Heavy	40% (use .40)

Age-adjusted BMR X (Percent of Activity level) = Activity Factor;

Age-adjusted BMR PLUS Activity factor = **DCA**

Examples:
1. Susan   gender: female
                                 weight: 135
                                 age: 25
                                 activity level: heavy
Step A: 135 X 11 = 1485 (BMR)
Step C: 1485 X .30 = 446
         1485 + 446 = 1931 (DCA)

2. James   gender: male
                                 weight: 220
                                 age: 67
                                 activity level: light
Step A: 220 X 12 = 2640 (BMR)
Step B: 2640 X .08 = 211
         2640 − 211 = 2429 (age-adjusted BMR)
Step C: 2429 X .15 = 364
         2429 + 364 = 2793 (DCA)

Appendix **L**

Reference Daily Intakes (RDI)*

Vitamin A	5,000	IU
Thiamin (B1)	1.5	mg
Riboflavin (B2)	1.7	mg
Niacin (B3)	20	mg
Vitamin B6	2	mg
Vitamin B12	6	mcg
Vitamin C	60	mg
Vitamin D	400	IU
Vitamin E	30	IU
Biotin	0.3	mg
Copper	2	mg
Folate (Folic Acid)	0.4	mg
Calcium	1,000	mg
Iodine	150	mcg
Iron	18	mg
Magnesium	400	mg
Pantothenic Acid	10	mg
Phosphorus	1,000	mg
Zinc	15	mg
Protein:		
5 years to adults	50	g
Pregnant Women	60	g
Nursing Mothers	65	g
Infants under 1 year	14	g
Children, 1 to 4 years	16	g

IU – international units   mg – milligrams
mcg – micrograms   g – grams

*For food labeling purposes, vitamins and minerals in the RDI are the same for all caloric levels, except for protein intake in certain populations. The listing of thiamine, riboflavin, and niacin in food labels are purely voluntary. These are no longer considered significant nutritional deficiencies.

Appendix M

Calculate Your Daily Carbohydrate, Protein, and Fat Allowances

Carbohydrate = 4 calories per gram
Protein = 4 calories per gram
Fat = 9 calories per gram

Data needed: Your Daily Caloric Allowance(DCA)

The following calculation is based on the following assumptions:
➤ Carbohydrate allowance is 60% of DCA
➤ Protein allowance is 10% of DCA
➤ Fat allowance is 30% of DCA

Formulas:

1. Carbohydrate Allowance:
DCA X .60 = 60% of total Calories
60% of Calories DIVIDED BY 4 = Daily Carbohydrate
Allowance

Example: If your DCA is 2,000
2,000 X .60 = 1,200 Calories
1,200 DIVIDED BY 4 = 300 g (Daily Carbohydrate
Allowance)

2. Protein Allowance:

DCA X .10 = 10% of total Calories

10% Calories DIVIDED BY 4 = Daily Protein Allowance

Example: If your DCA is 2,000

2,000 X .10 = 200 Calories

200 DIVIDED BY 4 = 50 g (Daily Protein Allowance)

3. Fat Allowance:

DCA X .30 = 30% of total Calories

30% Calories DIVIDED BY 9 = Daily Fat Allowance

Example: If your DCA is 2,000

2,000 X .30 = 600 Calories

600 DIVIDED BY 9 = 65 g (Daily Fat Allowance)

Use the same formula when you want to increase or lower the percentage of each nutrient. Just change the percentage number. Keep in mind that fat has a different amount of calories per gram as compared to carbohydrate and protein.

If you do not know your specific Daily Caloric Allowance (DCA), go to Appendix K, pages 262-263, for the calculation. Otherwise, you can go to Chapter 7, page 130, for the standardized DCA.

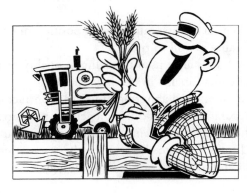

GLOSSARY

Acidophilus - A bacteria used in fermenting yogurt which is also found in the intestinal flora. It keep fungus and other harmful bacteria from proliferating.

Anti-angiogenesis - Ability to prevent the growth of blood vessels.

Carcinogen - A substance that can cause cancer.

Cyanosis - Bluish discoloration of the skin due to lack of oxygen.

Desquamation - shedding of the skin.

Diabetes mellitus - A carbohydrate metabolism disorder characterized by inadequate supply or utilization of insulin resulting to high blood sugar.

Dialysis - The separation of substances in solution by means of their unequal diffusion through semipermeable membranes.

Dyspnea - Difficulty in breathing.

Emesis - Act of vomiting.

Gastroenteritis - Inflammation of the stomach or intestine, usually associated with intolerance to food or foods.

Humectant - A substance that has the ability to retain moisture

Malaise - A vague sense of debility or ill-health.

Mutagen - A substance that can cause a change in the hereditary material of cells.

Myalgia - Muscle pain.

Myasthenia gravis - a disorder of the nueromuscular function characterized by progressive fatigue and exhasution of voluntary muscles.

Myelin - A covering of fatty material that encloses the nerve fibers of the body.

Neurologic - Pertaining to the nervous system, its disorders and treatments.

Prostration - The act of assuming a lying position due to exhaustion and lack of vitality or will to rise.

Sequestrant - A substance used to maintain quality of food by preventing metal contaminants in causing rancidity.

Spastic - Involuntary and abnormal muscular contraction.

Syneresis - Separation of liquid from a gel due to contraction.

Toxicity - The condition of being harmful or poisonous.

Vertigo - A disordered state characterized by a sensation of rotation or whirling of an individual or his surroundings.

REFERENCES

Addleman, Frank G. *The Winning Edge: Nutrition For Athletic Fitness and Performance.* New York: Prentice Hall Press, 1987.

American Council on Exercise. *Lifestyle and Weight Management:Consultant Manual.* Ed.. Richard T. Cotton. San Diego: ACE, 1996.

American Dietetic Association'.s *Food and Nutrition Guide, The.* Ed. Roberta Larson Duyff. Minneapolis: Chronimed Publishing, 1996.

Arnot, Bob. *The Breast Cancer Prevention Diet: The Powerful Foods, Supplements, And Drugs That Can Save Your Life.* New York: Little, Brown & Company, 1998.

Arnot, Bob. *Revolutionary Weight Control Program.* New York: Little, Brown & Company, 1997.

Balch, James F. and Phyllis A. *Prescription For Nutritional Healing.* Garden City Park: Avery Publishing Group, 1997.

Beling, Stephanie. *Power Foods.* New York: HarperCollins Publishers, Inc., 1997.

Brody, Jane E. *Jane Brody's Nutrition Book: A Lifetime Guide To Good Eating For Better Health And Weight Control.* New York: Bantam Books, 1988.

Bruce, Lowell K. *Mid-Life Body Signals.* New York: HarperCollins Publishers, Inc., 1997.

Burkholz, Herbert. *The FDA Follies: An Alarming Look At Our Food and Drugs In The 1980's.* New York: Basic Books, 1994.

Burton Goldberg Group, The. *Alternative Medicine: The Definitive Guide.* Puyallup: Future Medicine Publishing, Inc., 1994.

Chevallier, Andrew. *The Encyclopedia of Medicinal Plants: A Practical Reference Guide To More Than 550 Key Medicinal Plants And Their Uses.* New York: DK Publishing, Inc., 1996.

Complete Home Medical Encyclopedia, *The Symptoms.* Ed. Sigmund Stephen Miller. London: Macmillan London Ltd., 1979.

Connor, Sonja L. and William E. *The New American Diet.* New York: Simon and Schuster, 1986.

Cooper, Kenneth. *Advanced Nutritional Therapies.* Nashville: Thomas Nelson, Inc., 1996.

Davis, Goode P., Jr. and Park, Edwards. *The Human Body, The Heart: A Living Pump.* New York: Torstar Books, Inc. 1984.

Dibb, Sue. *What The Label Doesn't Tell You.* Glasgow: Caledonian International Book Manufacturing, Ltd., 1997.

Dadd, Debra Lynn. *Non-Toxic and Natural.* Los Angeles: Jeremy P. Tarcher, Inc. 1984.

Duke, James A. *The Green Pharmacy.* New York: St Martin's Press, 1997.

Eades, Michael R. and Mary Dan. *Protein Power.* New York: Bantam Books, 1998.

Fletcher, Anne M. *Eating Thin For Life.* Shelburne: Chapters Publishing, Ltd., 1997.

Fox, Arnold. and Adderly, Brenda. *The Fat Blocker Diet.* New York: Affinity Communications Corp., 1997.

Freydberg, Nicholas and Gortner, Willis A. *The Food Additives Book.* Toronto: Bantam Books, 1982.

Gaesser, Glenn A. *Big Fat Lies: The Truth About Your Health.* New York: Ballantine Books, 1996.

Garrison, Robert, Jr. and Somer, Elizabeth. *The Nutrition Desk Reference.* New Canaan: Keats Publishing, 1985.

Gittleman, Ann Louise., *et al. Your Body Knows Best.* New York: Pocket Books. 1996.

Goldbeck, Nikki and David. *The Healthiest Diet In The World.* New york: Penguin Group, 1998.

Goldberg, Burton. *Alternative Medicine Guide to Heart Disease.* Tiburon: Future Medicine Publishing, 1997.

Haas, Robert. *Permanent Remissions.* New York: Pocket Books, 1997.

Hausman, Patricia and Hurley, Judith Benn. *The Healing Foods: The Ultimate Authority on The Curative Power of Nutrition.* Emmaus: Rodale Press, 1989.

Health Reference Series. *Diet & Nutrition Sourcebook, Volume XV.* Ed. Dan R. Harris. Detroit: Omnigraphics, 1996.

Heimlich, Jane. *What Your Doctor Won't Tell You.* New York: HarperCollins Publishers, 1990.

Heller, Richard F. and Rachael F. *The Carbohydrate Addict's Lifespan Program.* New York: Penguin Group, 1997

Lowell, Bruce K. *Mid-Life Body Signals.* New York: HarperCollins Publishers, Inc., 1997.

Marti, James E. and Blackburn, George L. *The Ultimate Consumer's Guide To Diets and Nutrition.* New York: Houghton Mifflin Company, 1997.

McCoy, Joseph J. *How Safe Is Our Food Supply?* New York: F. Watts, 1990.

Mindell, Earl. *Vitamin Bible.* New York: Warner Books, 1991.

Ministry of Agriculture, Fisheries and Food. *Manual Of Nutrition.* Eds. David Buss and Jean Robertson. London: Her Majesty's Stationery Office, 1984.

Mollen, Art. *Dr. Mollen's Anti-Aging Diet: The Breakthrough Program For Easy Weight Loss And Longevity.* New York, Penguin Books, 1992.

Murray, Michael and Pizzorno, Joseph. *Encyclopedia Of Natural Medicine.* Rocklin: Prima Publishing, 1991.

Netzer, Corinne T. *The Complete Book Of Food Counts.* New York: Dell Publishing, 1991.

Perucca, Fabien and Pouradier, Gerard. *The Rubbish On Our Plates.* Translation from French by Joe Laredo. London: Prior Books, 1996.

Prevention Magazine Health Books' Editors. *Food and Nutrition.* Ed. John Feltman. Emmaus: Rodale Press, Inc., 1993.

Pritikin, Nathan. *The Pritikin Promise: 28 Days To A Longer, Healthier Life.* New York: Bantam Books, Inc., 1985.

Ody, Penelope. *The Complete Medicinal Herbal: A Practical Guide To The Healing Properties Of Herbs, With More Than 250 Remedies For Common Ailments.* New York: Doring Kindersley, Inc., 1993.

Reader's Digest, The. *Eat Better, Live Better: A Commonsense Guide to Nutrition and Good health.* Ed. Joseph L. Gardner. Pleasantville: The Reader's Digest Association, Inc., 1982.

Reader's Digest, The. *Foods That Harm, Foods That Heal. Pleasantville:* The Reader's Digest Association, Inc., 1997.

Rinzler, Carol Ann. *Nutrition For Dummies.* Foster City: IDG Books Worldwide, Inc.,1997.

Sears, Barry. *Enter The Zone.* New York: HarperCollins Publisher, Inc, 1995.

Shyrock, Harold. *You And Your Health, Volume I.* Mountainview: Pacific Press Publishing Association, 1979.
Shyrock, Harold. *You And Your health, Volume II.* Mountainview: Pacific Press Publishing Association, 1979.

Shyrock, Harold. *You and Your Health, Volume III.* Mountainview: Pacific Press Publishing Association, 1979.

Sonberg, Lynn. *The Health Nutrient Bible.* New York: Simon & Schuster, Inc., 1995.

Spiller, Gene. *The Super Pyramid Eating Program.* New York: Times Books, 1993.

Steinman, David. *Diet For A Poisoned Planet: How To Choose Safe Foods For You And Your Family.* New York: Ballantine Books, 1992.

Steinman, David. and Epstein, Samuel S. *The Safe Shopper's Bible: A Consumer's Guide To Nontoxic Household Products, Cosmetics, and Food.* New York: MacMillan, Inc., 1995.

Steinman, David and Wisner, Michael R. *Living Healthy In A Toxic World.* New York: The Berkley Publishing Group, 1996.

Turner, Lisa. *Meals That Heal: A Nutraceutical Approach To Diet and Health.* Rochester: Healing Arts Press, 1996.
Wargo, John. *Our Children's Toxic Legacy: How Science And Law Fail To Protect Us from Pesticides.* New Haven: Yale University Press, 1996.

Weil, Andrew. *Healthy Living.* New York: Ballantine Books, 1997.

West, Edward Staunton, *et al. Textbook of Bichemistry.* New York: The Macmillan Company, 1968.

INDEX

About the Authors:

Nancy G. Balingasa is a B.A. graduate with diplomas in Fitness and Nutrition, and in Medical Transcription. Manager of a training center for community development workers in Southeast Asia, she also worked as Training Consultant in East Africa. She is a certified Personal Trainor and has been an Exercise Instructor for more than fifteen years. Her writing experience consists of editorial work, feature writing, training manuals, and references.

Eduardo N. Balingasa holds an M.Sc. degree in Agronomy, specialized in Plant Breeding and Genetics. He was Consultant to the United Nations Development Programme (UNDP) in Southeast Asia and worked as Agricultural Expert with the German Agency for Technical Cooperation (GTZ) in East Africa. He has authored and co-authored a number of scientific publications, research manuals, and other technical references.

Notice to Readers

We hope that this book will help you to have better health and a happier life. Should that happen, the efforts we exerted to make this book available to you will not have been wasted.

We will be updating this book when new knowledge comes along. If you have any questions or opinions to share, we would be pleased to hear from you.

Contact Nancy or Ed Balingasa at:

Printed Matters
114 Sage Blue Court
The Woodlands, Texas 77382-1347

Telephone: (409) 273-2943
FAX: (409) 273-6943
email: info@printedmatters.com
http:// www.printedmatters.com

THE FOOD JUNGLE
Order Form

makes a great gift!

No. of Copies_____X $14.95 per copy $ _____
Sales Tax: (8.25% Texas residents only)   _____
Shipping & Handling ($4.00 per copy)   _____

TOTAL $ ==============

Ordered By:
Name:_____
Address: _____
City:_____State: _____
ZipCode:_____Daytime Phone:_____

Ship To: (*If different than "Ordered By"*)
Name:_____
Address: _____
City:_____State: _____
ZipCode:_____Daytime Phone:_____

Method of Payment:
( ) **Check or Money Order***
( ) **Credit Card:****   ( ) Visa   ( ) Mastercard
                ( ) Discover   ( ) American Express
Card Number:_____Exp.Date:_____
Signature Required: _____

*Mail this form and payment to:
Printed matters
114 Sage Blue Court
The Woodlands, TX 77382-1347

**Phone: (888) 273-3155